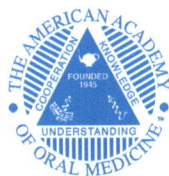

CLINICIAN'S GUIDE
Diagnosis and Treatment of
Chronic Orofacial Pain
FOURTH EDITION

EDITORS

Shawn S. Adibi, DDS, MEd
Associate Professor, Department of
General Practice and Dental Public
Health, The University of Texas School
of Dentistry at Houston

Istvan A. Hargitai, DDS, MS
Chairman, Specialty Leader
Navy Orofacial Pain
Naval Postgraduate Dental School
Bethesda, MD

Charles S. Greene, DDS
Clinical Professor
Department of Orthodontics
UIC College of Dentistry

Pamela J. Gardner, DMD
Chief, Dental Consult Service
National Institute of Dental and
Craniofacial Research
Bethesda, MD

CONTRIBUTING AUTHORS

Kenneth Abramovitch, DDS, MS
Shawn S. Adibi, DDS, MEd
Robert N. Arm, DMD
B. Antonia Balciunas, DDS,MSD
Bruce Blasberg, DDS
Ronald S. Brown, DDS, MS
Jerry E. Bouquot DDS, MSD
Sharon L. Brooks, DDS, MS
Jeffrey A. Burgess, DDS, MSD
Glenn T. Clark, DDS, MS
Joel B. Epstein, DMD, MSD
Pamela J. Gardner, DMD
Jean-Paul Goulet, DDS, MSD
Martin S. Greenberg, DDS
Charles S. Greene, DDS
Miriam Grushka, DDS, PhD
Istvan A. Hargitai, DDS, MS
Wayne W. Herman, DDS,MS
Barry Hinderstein, DDS, PhD
Joseph L. Konzelman, DDS
Gilles J. Lavigne, DMD, MSc
Benoit LaLonde, DMD, MSD
Craig S. Miller, DDS, MS
Michael A. Siegel, DDS, MS
David Sirois, DMD, PhD
Thomas P. Sollecito, DMD

Contributing authors are members
of the American Academy of Oral
Medicine. This monograph represents a
consensus of the contributing authors
and not necessarily the private views of
any of the individuals

CONTENTS

American Academy of Oral Medicine
2150 N. 107th St., Suite 205
Seattle, Washington 98133
TEL: (206) 209-5279
EMAIL: info@aaom.com   WEBSITE: www.aaom.com
©2017 American Academy of Oral Medicine

Notice

The authors and publisher have made every effort to ensure that the patient care recommended herein, including choice of drugs and drug dosages, is in accord with the accepted standard and practice at the time of publication. However, since research and regulation constantly change clinical standards, the reader is urged to check the product information sheet included in the package of each drug, which includes recommended doses, warnings, and contraindications. This is particularly important with new or infrequently used drugs. Any treatment regimen, particularly one involving medication, involves inherent risk that must be weighed on a case-by-case basis against the benefits anticipated. The reader is cautioned that the purpose of this book is to inform and enlighten; the information contained herein is not intended as, and should not be employed as, a substitute for individual diagnosis and treatment.

ISBN
print: 978-1-936176-45-8
PDF: 978-1-936176-46-5
EPUB: 978-1-936176-47-2
Kindle: 978-1-936176-48-9

Printed in the United States

The fourth edition of this Guide is dedicated to the memory of Jonathan A. Ship, DMD. Dr. Ship was an inspiration to a generation of students, oral medicine residents and colleagues and a revered member of the American Academy of Oral Medicine. His research contributions in geriatric dentistry, Xerostomia, Sjögren's syndrome and oral, head and neck cancer will serve the professional community and society for generations. His friendship, guidance, professionalism and laughter are sorely missed by everyone who knew and loved him. Dr. Ship has contributed extensively to this Guide.

ABOUT THE AMERICAN ACADEMY OF ORAL MEDICINE (AAOM): The AAOM is a 501c6; nonprofit organization founded in 1945 as the American Academy of Dental Medicine and took its current name in 1966. The members of the American Academy of Oral Medicine include an internationally recognized group of health care professionals and experts concerned with the oral health care of patients who have complex medical conditions, oral mucosal disorders, and / or chronic orofacial pain. Oral Medicine is the field of dentistry concerned with the oral health care of medically complex patients and with the diagnosis and non-surgical management of medically-related disorders or conditions affecting the oral and maxillofacial region.

AMERICAN ACADEMY OF
ORAL MEDICINE

MISSION:

1. To promote the study and dissemination of knowledge of the medical aspects of dentistry while serving the best interests of the public.

2. To promote the highest standards of care in the diagnosis and treatment of oral conditions that are not responsive to conventional dental or oral maxillofacial surgical procedures.

3. To provide an avenue of referral for dental practitioners who have patients with severe, life- threatening medical disorders or complex diagnostic problems involving the oral and maxillofacial region that require ongoing nonsurgical management.

4. To improve the quality of life of patients with medically related oral disease.

5. To foster increased understanding and cooperation between medical and dental professions.

6. To obtain American Dental Association recognition of oral medicine as a specialty.

The Academy achieves these goals by holding national meetings annually; by presenting lectures, workshops, and seminars; by sponsorship of the American Board of Oral Medicine; by the editorship of the Oral Medicine Section of *Oral Surgery, Oral Medicine, Oral Pathology, Oral Radiology*, and *Endodontics*; and by publishing monographs and position papers on timely subjects relating to oral medicine.

This Clinician's Guide is another AAOM educational service.
Other Clinician's Guides available from the Academy include:

Treatment of Common Oral Conditions,
7/e Tobacco Cessation
Oral Health in Geriatric Patients, 3/e
Pharmacology, 2/e
Medically Complex Dental Patients 4/e
Salivary Gland & Chemosensory Disorders 1/e

Preface

Thank you for the purchase of the AAOM *Clinician's Guide to Diagnosis and Treatment of Chronic Orofacial Pain*. This publication is the culmination of a great deal of work from a wide array of authors, including a number of world leaders and widely recognized educators in their respective areas of contribution. This Monograph originally developed by wide array of renowned clinicians listed in editor's page. It represents the consensus of experts within leadership of AAOM. Readers are to exercise clinical judgments in context of the clinical findings and circumstances and with respect to the local and state laws. The diagnosis of orofacial and odontogenic pain is often complicated and perplexing. Patients may experience pain in a particular tooth for no apparent reason and not experience pain in an obviously diseased tooth. As dentists, we tend to focus on the hard structures of tooth and bone, with less attention to soft tissues such as muscle, blood vessels, nerves, and connective tissue. Chronic orofacial pain requires a broader base of understanding and comprehensive assessment. In the past, clinicians' attempts to shape our view of chronic orofacial pain to be consistent with hard tissue pathology may have colored the paradigm. The aim of this guide is to promote a more comprehensive, reasonable, logical model of chronic orofacial pain.

The diagnosis and treatment of chronic orofacial pain conditions are often difficult tasks. Time, effort, experience, and education are required. At present, there are gaps within our scientific knowledge base concerning etiology, diagnosis, and therapies of all of the chronic pain conditions. Controlled scientific studies may not exist for many of these conditions. Therefore, the state of the art is determined by both science and the art of patient management. We must rely on science whenever possible; in the absence of science, we are left to consensus of opinions, the teachings of others, and clinical judgment.

The primary goal of the dentist/clinician who sees a patient suffering with pain should be to establish a diagnosis. The clinician must understand the mechanisms and behavioral aspects of pain. It should always be remembered that it is just as important to rule out a problem as it is to identify it. The clinician is responsible for establishing a differential diagnosis because at times the diagnostic process must rely on the process of elimination. It is of vital importance that treatment be based on diagnosis. Treatment without diagnosis is careless and potentially dangerous, and diagnosis without treatment is an empty effort.

The aim of this guide is to provide an aid and overview for general dentists for the assessment, diagnosis, and treatment of chronic orofacial pain. Readers may wish to begin with the appendices for an overview of the patient workup and evaluation. Because of the complexity of the subject, a work of this size cannot cover in detail the numerous conditions that are included. It is hoped that the simplified format will aid the clinician in the treatment of the orofacial pain patient with respect to differential diagnoses and current therapies. More comprehensive references are listed at the end of this guide. The views expressed in this guide represent a consensus and are not necessarily the views of individual contributors.

Readers are strongly encouraged to review references listed at the end of this monograph and expand their knowledge and skills on desired subject matter of their choice. Once again, thank you for the purchase of the AAOM *Clinician's Guide to Diagnosis and Treatment of Chronic Orofacial Pain*. We hope that it is a useful addition to your reference library and welcome suggestions for alterations and additions that may be incorporated into future editions.

Shawn Adibi, *Editors-in-Chief*

Acknowledgement

The contributions of Drs. William N. Alexander, Ralph I. Brooke, Harold Merskey, and Richard D. Riva, Academy co-authors of the first edition, are greatly appreciated.

Standard Abbreviations

I	One	Prn	as needed (pro re nata)
ii	Two	Q	Every
iii	Three	q2h	every 2 hours
a	Before	q4h	every 4 hours
ac	before meals (ante cibum)	q6h	every 6 hours
ad lib	as desired (ad libitum)	q8h	every 8 hours
asap	as soon as possible	q12h	every 12 hours
AAOM	American Academy of Oral Medicine	Qam	every morning
bid	twice a day (bis in die)	Qd	every day (quaque die)
btl	Bottle	Qhs	every bedtime
c	With	Qid	four times a day (quarter in die)
cap	Capsule	Qod	every other day
CBC	complete blood count	Qpm	every evening
CDC	U. S. Center for Disease Control and Prevention	qsad	add a sufficient quantity to equal
crm	Cream	qwk	every week
disp	dispense on a prescription label	RAS	recurrent aphthous stomatitis
elix	Elixir	RAU	recurrent aphthous ulcer
FDA	U.S. Food and Drug Administration	RBC	red blood cell count
g	Gram	RHL	recurrent herpes labialis
gtt	Drop	RIH	recurrent intraoral herpes
h	Hour	Rx	Prescription
hs	at bedtime	s	Without
HSV	herpes simplex virus	Sig	patient dosing instructions on prescription label
IU	international units	Sol	Solution
IV	Intravenous	SPF	sun protection factor
L	Liter	stat	Immediately
liq	Liquid	Syr	Syrup
loz	Lozenge	Tab	Tablet
Mg	Milligram	tbsp	Tablespoon
Min	Minute	Tid	three times a day (ter in die)
mL	Milliliter	Top	Topical
NaF	sodium fluoride	Tsp	Teaspoon

Standard Abbreviations (continued)

Oint	Ointment	U	Unit
OTC	over-the-counter	ut dict	as directed (ut dictum)
Oz	Ounce	UV	Ultraviolet
P	After	Visc	Viscous
Pc	after meals	VZV	varicella-zoster virus
PABA	para-aminobenzoic acid	WBC	white blood cell count
PHN	postherpetic neuralgia	Wk	Week
PLT	platelet count	Yr	Year
Po	by mouth (per os)	Zn	Zinc

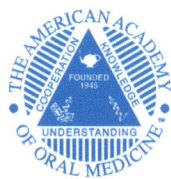

1 Oral Neuropathic Pain Conditions

Neuritis, neuralgia, neuropathy, and neuroma are specific entities that have a common characteristic—pain. As pain is always subjective, the differential diagnosis may be difficult and the management challenging. Conditions such as temporal arteritis, sympathetically maintained pain, and deep somatic pain may be related to these entities. As with all physical problems, a complete history, a careful clinical examination, and the proper use of diagnostic modalities are imperative.

NEURITIS

Neuritis denotes an inflammatory process that involves a nerve. In the oral and facial regions, the most common causes include trauma, infection, and viral disorders (see Table 1–1).

GENERAL CHARACTERISTICS:
- No trigger zone
- No autonomic signs
- No motor signs
- Deep pain/burning

OUTCOME: The prognosis is generally favorable but depends on the patient's ability to tolerate the therapeutic procedures. In difficult cases, referral may be indicated (i.e., to prosthodontics, oral and maxillofacial surgery).

NEURALGIA

The International Association for the Study of Pain (IASP) currently defines neuralgia as pain in the distribution of one or more nerves. The neuralgias of greatest interest to the dentist are typical neuralgias (trigeminal neuralgia and glossopharyngeal neuralgia), atypical neuralgia/ atypical facial pain (see Chapter 2, "Atypical Facial Pain (Persistent Facial Pain of Unknown Etiology)"), and postherpetic neuralgia.

Typical Neuralgias

The so-called typical neuralgias have some elements in common, such as sharp, stabbing, lancinating pain, following nerve pathways, and having the ability to be physically stimulated (triggered).

GENERAL CHARACTERISTICS:
- Paroxysmal (sudden attack)
- Both male and female
- Follows nerve distribution
- Extremely intense
- Hyperalgesia/ allodynia
- Pain intensity disproportionate
- Paresthesia
- Shocking or electric-like
- Anesthesia
- Presence of a refractory period
- Presence of a trigger zone
- No referred pain or autonomic signs
- Usually after age 50 years (if < age 40 years, rule out multiple sclerosis)
- Local/ topical anesthesia may arrest trigger points

TABLE 1–1: MENTAL NERVE COMPRESSION		
General Characteristics	*Population Dynamics*	*Treatment*
Pain when chewing	Elderly female	Denture adjustment, soft liner
Pain while wearing dentures	Alveolar atrophy/cachectic	Bone graft/new dentures
Pain relief by removing dentures	Osteoporosis	Implant/prosthetics

Trigeminal Neuralgia (Tic Douloureux)

This neuralgia of the trigeminal or fifth cranial nerve is triggered and produces a sharp, superficial pain likened to an electric shock; it can last seconds and up to 2 minutes, with pain-free intervals. Precipitating factors include touching or stroking of the trigger-point area and air currents. The most common nerve distribution affected is the mandibular division (V3) of the trigeminal nerve, although it also can occur in V1 and V2. The above description is termed classic trigeminal neuralgia and there may be imaging evidence of vascular compression of the trigeminal nerve root at the pons, or it may be idiopathic. The term secondary trigeminal neuralgia is reserved for impingements due to other lesions. Mimickers of trigeminal neuralgia may be seen in patients with disorders such as multiple sclerosis. Occasionally it may occur with cluster headaches (cluster-tic syndrome).

GENERAL CHARACTERISTICS:
- Trigger zone (to innocuous stimuli)
- Sharp electric-like pain
- Unilateral
- Lasts seconds to minutes
- Pain-free intervals (refractory period)
- Pain may induce facial muscle contraction (tic)
- V3 > V2 > V1

SWEET CRITERIA: (*consider including SWEET and/or ICHD criteria*)
- Pain is paroxysmal
- Provoked by light touch to face (trigger zones)
- Confined to trigeminal distribution
- Unilateral
- Clinical exam is normal

INTERNATIONAL CLASSIFICATION OF HEADACHE DISORDERS CRITERIA (3rd edition, ß version)
- At least three attacks of unilateral facial pain fulfilling the following criteria:
- Occurring in one or more divisions of the trigeminal nerve, with no radiation beyond the trigeminal distribution
- Pain has at least three of the following 4 characteristics:
    1. recurring in paroxysmal attacks lasting from a fraction of a second to 2 minutes
    2. severe intensity
    3. electric shock-like, shooting, stabbing or sharp in quality
    4. precipitated by innocuous stimuli to the affected side of the face
- No clinically evident neurological deficit and not better accounted for by another diagnosis

Neuralgia-Inducing Cavitational Osteonecrosis

Neuralgia-inducing Cavitational Osteonecrosis continues to represent a controversial diagnosis within the oral and maxillofacial complex. It is an established entity within long bones, however. Some researchers and clinicians believe that a nonspecific infection manifests within bone cavities in the jaws and elicits neuropathic pain. Therefore, these clinicians propose anesthetic localization to define the location of the lesions and surgical treatment to enucleate the infected bone cavities. Many other clinicians and researchers believe that this entity has not been adequately demonstrated as a diagnostic entity within the head and neck region. Presently, accepted diagnostic criteria and therapeutic regimens have not been established.

MANAGEMENTS FOR NEURALGIAS: The role of the dentist is essentially to rule out pain of odontogenic origin and refer to clinicians experienced in the management of neuropathic pain. It is important that unnecessary dental procedures not be performed. The dentist must have an accurate diagnosis before proceeding with irreversible treatment such as endodontic or surgical procedures. Unnecessary interventions delay appropriate therapy and have the potential to negatively impact upon the pain complaint.

POSSIBLE MANAGEMENTS BY SPECIALISTS
- Anticonvulsant drug therapy (centrally acting pain medications)
- Surgical decompression
- Neurolysis/radiofrequency (RF) / alcohol injection / stereotactic radiosurgery (Gamma Knife®)
- Neurolysis/rhizotomy
- Nerve sectioning

OUTCOME: The prognosis varies. Drug therapy (i.e., carbamazepine, phenytoin, lamotrigine, baclofen, etc.) is often effective, and surgery is reserved for those who do not achieve adequate pain control or experience severe side effects from medical management. For those who require neurosurgical care, 70 to 90% have a 3- to 10-year success rate with microvascular decompression, although other therapeutic modalities are successful in many instances. Comparative outcomes of alcohol block, neurectomy, and RF thermocoagulation are as follows: RF, 83%; neurectomy, 51%; and alcohol block, 42%, with 8-year satisfactory relief, but all are associated with individual failures ranging from 49 to 84%.

Glossopharyngeal Neuralgia

Glossopharyngeal neuralgia is a rare condition that affects the glossopharyngeal or ninth cranial nerves and involves the posterior lateral portion of the tongue and the tonsillar pillar and surrounding pharyngeal mucosa. It may produce radiating pain to the ear and neck.

GENERAL CHARACTERISTICS:
- Paroxysmal—sudden onset, brief
- 50 years of age or more usually
- Triggered by swallowing, chewing, or coughing
- Usually unilateral, burning in character
- Males affected more often than females
- Posterior or oral pharyngeal areas
- Topical anesthetic spray to tonsillar fossa for diagnostic test (produces temporary remission)

INTERNATIONAL CLASSIFICATION OF HEADACHE DISORDERS CRITERIA (3rd edition, ß version)
- At least three attacks of unilateral pain fulfilling the following criteria:
- Pain is located in the posterior part of the tongue, tonsillar fossa, pharynx, beneath the angle of the lower jaw and/or in the ear
- Pain has at least 3 of the following 4 characteristics:
  1. recurring in paroxysmal attacks lasting from a few seconds to 2 minutes
  2. severe intensity
  3. shooting, stabbing or sharp in quality
  4. precipitated by swallowing, coughing, talking or yawning
- No clinically evident neurological deficit and not better accounted for by another diagnosis.

MANAGEMENTS: See Trigeminal Neuralgia.

OUTCOME: The prognosis varies. Surgical sectioning of the ninth nerve is the most effective treatment, although spontaneous remission may occur (see also Trigeminal Neuralgia).

Herpes Zoster and Postherpetic Neuralgia

Herpes zoster is the result of reactivation of latent varicella zoster virus (VZV). A previous history of chickenpox may be helpful in the early recognition of this condition. The lay term for this disease process is shingles. Postherpetic neuralgia may occur after an outbreak of VZV.

GENERAL CHARACTERISTICS:
- Severe burning pain with or without observable lesions
- Follows the distribution of the trigeminal nerve in the orofacial type
- Itching
- Intraoral and/or extra-oral lesions
- Unilateral dermatomal distribution; rarely crosses the midline
- Lesions when observed may be crusting or vesiculoerosive
- May also affect the thoracic area
- 80% spinal and 20% trigeminal nerve involvement

DIAGNOSIS: The diagnosis of herpes zoster prior to the occurrence of skin or mucosal lesions may be difficult. However, the earlier the diagnosis is made, the more effective is the treatment. Postherpetic neuralgia may produce severe pain for months or years. VZV and postherpetic neuralgia are found most frequently in individuals after 50 years of age. This condition may be associated with immunocompromised patients such as those with diabetes, leukemia, lymphoma, and human immunodeficiency virus/acquired immune deficiency syndrome (HIV/AIDS).

MANAGEMENTS:
- Rule out dental causes
- Palliative therapies
- Refer to Oral Medicine (trial drug therapy; see below)*
- Refer to a physician (i.e., internal medicine, infectious diseases)

Palliative therapies include cocoa butter ointment and lanolin-based lip preparations, or petrolatum as an emollient may be palliative. Patients must wash their hands frequently and should be advised of the infectious nature of this process.

For Herpes Zoster (VZV):

Rx: Acyclovir (Zovirax) 800 mg capsules
Disp: 50 capsules
Sig: Take 1 capsule five times daily as close to the prodromal stage as possible.

Rx: Valacyclovir (Valtrex) 500 mg capsules
Disp: 80 capsules
Sig: Take 4 capsules three times daily as close to the prodromal stage as possible.

Rx: Famciclovir (Famvir) 500 mg capsules
Disp: 21 capsules
Sig: Take 1 capsule three times daily for 7 days starting as close to the prodromal stage as possible.

* Systemic steroids have been employed to ameliorate this condition. However, the use of these pharmacotherapeutics is not recommended by clinicians without experience with steroids. Referral is suggested to Oral Medicine or a physician with experience in the use of steroids.

For Postherpetic Neuralgia (Tricyclic Antidepressant Therapy):

> **Rx**: Amitriptyline 10 or 25 mg tablets
> Disp: 40 tablets
> Sig: Take 1 tablet hs.

> **Rx**: Nortriptyline 10 mg or 25 mg tablets
> Disp: 40 tablets
> Sig: Take 1 tablet hs.

After 4 weeks (if there is no perceived benefit), increase the dosage by one 25 mg tablet (or 10 mg tablet) and 4 weeks later (if there is still no perceived benefit) by one more 25 mg tablet (up to 75 mg per day) depending on the patient's tolerance of the medication. Tricyclic antidepressants (TCAs) may need 2 to 3 weeks before they become effective in relieving pain. TCAs are known to cause some drowsiness initially or on increasing the dosage regimen. Further, they are known to cause xerostomia and have other known side effects. Patients should be informed of the increased risk of dental decay with xerostomia. In addition to frequent dental checkups, recommend increased oral hygiene effort, reduction of cariogenic diet, and daily topical fluoride treatment (ie. Prevident). After continued pain relief, the dosage should be titrated down and discontinued. Other TCAs, such as doxepin and desipramine, are also effective in the treatment of chronic pain.

Antiseizure Drugs for the Treatment of Chronic Pain:

> **Rx**: Gabapentin 600 mg scored tablets
> Disp: 50 tablets
> Sig: Day 1: ½ tablet; Day 2: ½ tablet bid; Day 3: ½ tablet tid.
>   Maintain for 2 weeks; dosage may be titrated up to 3
>   tablets tid.

Substance P Depleter:

> **Rx**: Capsaicin (Zostrix) crm 0.025% or 0.075%
> Disp: 1 tube
> Sig: Apply a small dab to the skin of affected area tid or qid*.

* Intraoral use should be limited to oral medicine clinicians.

Systemic steroids may be useful in treatment of VZV infection and may be helpful in ameliorating secondary post zoster neuralgia. Referral to a clinician skilled in the use of these medications is suggested.

OUTCOME: Postherpetic neuralgia sometimes begins long after the infection (VZV) has subsided. This condition occasionally undergoes spontaneous resolution. Immediate referral to an oral medicine clinician or a physician with early intervention may improve the prognosis. High-dose antiviral therapy should be considered during episodes of clinical infection but is of no benefit for postherpetic neuralgia. (Refer to above or to *Clinician's Guide to Treatment of Common Oral Conditions, 7th Edition*)

NEUROMA

Neuroma is a benign tumor of nerve origin that develops following surgical procedures or trauma. It is made up largely of nerve cells and nerve fibers. Neuromas are often given specific names based on the predominant cell type or fiber (i.e., neurilemma derived from the Schwann cells of the myelin sheath). True neuromas are rarely a cause of orofacial pain. The traumatic neuroma (not a true tumor), however, tends to be painful and is a reactive, disorganized nerve bundle resulting from either accidental or iatrogenic damage, usually affecting a peripheral nerve.

GENERAL CHARACTERISTICS:
- Painful area readily localized by patient
- Pain exacerbated by dentures in the edentulous patient
- Localized pain, particularly in an area of previous surgery or injection
- Topical anesthetic does not relieve pain
- Area painful to palpation
- Pain exacerbated by mechanical stimulation (i.e., chewing)
- Injection of local anesthetic into the area relieves pain
- Most frequent in adults
- Also found in soft tissue of lip, tongue, or buccal mucosa

MANAGEMENTS:
- Refer to Oral Medicine for medical intervention
- Refer to Oral and Maxillofacial Surgery
- Refer to Neurology/Neurosurgery
- Early treatment improves outcome.

PAIN OF SOMATIC ORIGIN

Pain may emanate from somatic structures such as muscle, blood vessels, and teeth.

Deep Somatic Pain

In the head and neck region, the major categories of deep somatic pain include (1) tooth pain, (2) Musculoskeletal pain, (3) vascular pain, (4) maxillary sinusitis, and (5) head and neck and central nervous system cancer (also see Chapter 4, "Temporomandibular Disorders: Myogenous and Arthrogenous Conditions," for somatic muscular pain). Referred pain from outside the head and neck region, such as referred cardiac pain, may mimic deep somatic pain. Although headaches are a common cause of deep somatic pain, the diagnosis and management of headache are beyond the scope of this monograph (refer to The American Academy of Orofacial Pain listed in reference).

GENERAL CHARACTERISTICS:

- Pain intensity ranges from mild to severe
- Usually aching—dull, depressing
- Autonomic and motor signs are common
- May be described as shooting or radiating at times
- Mode of onset is usually induced but may be spontaneous
- The pain may be referred to other areas

Odontogenic Pain

Odontogenic disorders such as pulpitis, caries, dentinal sensitivity, Pericoronitis, cracked tooth syndrome, asymptomatic endodontic lesions, root fractures or clinical crown fractures, and periodontitis should not be overlooked as a potential cause for chronic orofacial pain. As these conditions may involve referred pain (site of the pain), the dentist is important in identifying these potential pain sources. Odontogenic disorders should be referred to a dental provider for appropriate diagnosis and therapy as indicated or to rule out an odontogenic cause of pain. Odontogenic causes as dentinal hypersensitivity secondary to tooth brush abrasion can cause moderate to severe chronic pain. (Suggested treatment includes a mechanical soft toothbrush, fluoride therapy, and desensitizing toothpastes or agents.)

Maxillary Sinusitis

Infection and inflammation of the maxillary sinuses are common. The location of the sinuses adjacent to the maxillary posterior teeth may result in pain referred to the dental structures and particularly the maxillary first molars and second bicuspids. Infected teeth may at times be the cause of maxillary sinusitis.

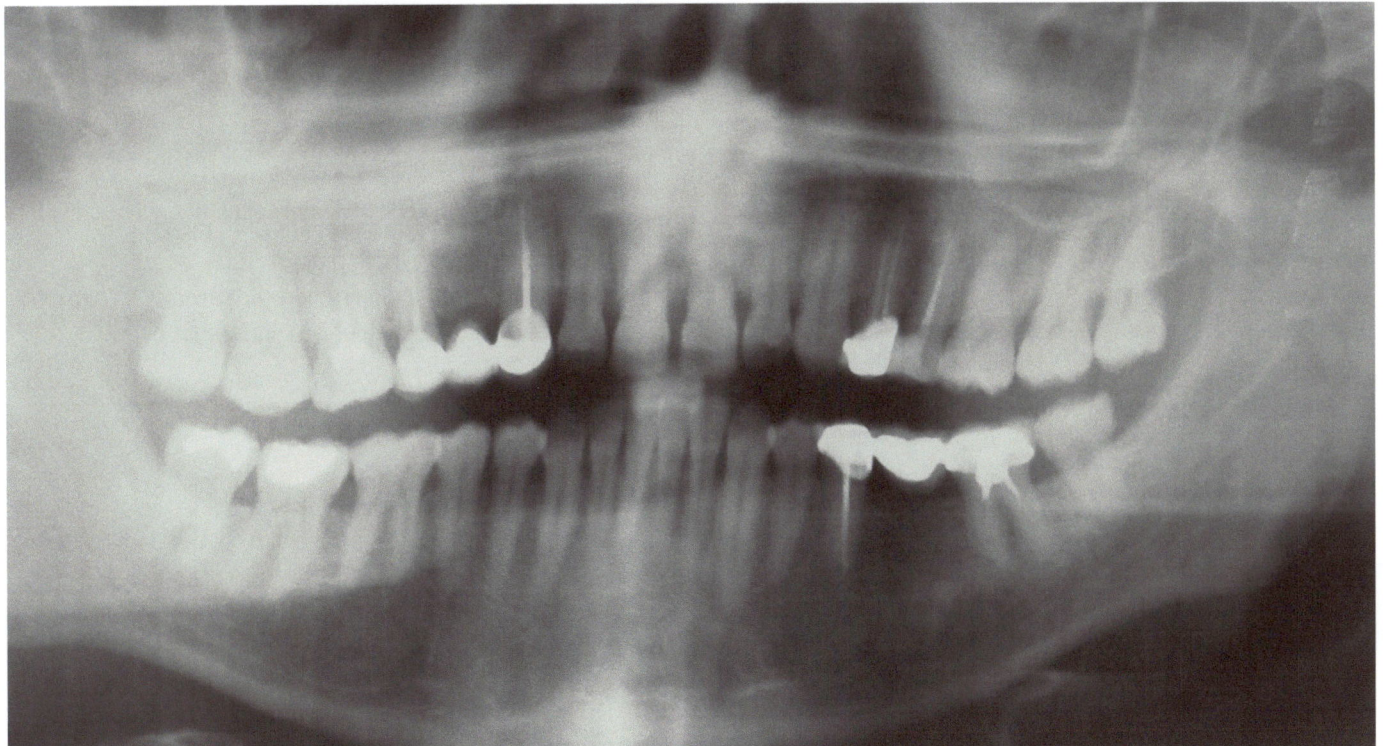

Figure 1-1: *Panoramic radiograph demonstrating chronic maxillary sinusitis, also see image provided in Appendix III*

GENERAL CLINICAL SYMPTOMATOLOGY:
- Stuffiness and maxillary pain during movements such as running or walking
- Changing the position of the head may influence the pain
- Runny nose and postnasal discharge may be present

GENERAL CLINICAL CHARACTERISTICS:
- Panoramic and/or dental radiographs may show abnormalities (Figure 1-1)
  - A. Cloudy sinus in acute cases
  - B. Thickened sinus floor in chronic sinusitis
- A Waters view film or computed tomography (CT) may show a fluid level and/or thickened sinus membrane
- Percussion of premolar and molar maxillary teeth reveals tenderness
- Teeth free of disease and vital
- Pressure applied to trigeminal infraorbital area elicits discomfort
- Medical history may indicate presence of chronic sinus problems and allergies or asthma

MANAGEMENTS:
- Rule out dental disease
- Refer to an otolaryngology specialist
- Interim or trial therapy may be initiated using OTC sinus medications such as antihistamines and decongestants (e.g., diphenhydramine)
- Antibiotics may be used after a definitive diagnosis of infection

OUTCOMES: The prognosis is good, although recurrence of sinusitis is common.

Vascular Pain

Vascular pain is pain owing to stimulation of somatic or autonomic sensory receptors or afferent fibers of arteries or perivascular tissues. This may be due to vessel dilation where the vessel walls are stretched and sensory receptors are stimulated. Local edema of the vessel wall and perivascular tissue and associated muscle pain may be involved. Conditions such as migraine, cluster headache, carotidynia, and temporal arteritis are examples of vascular pain. Possible etiologies include allergy, autoimmunity, and histamine release. These conditions usually occur in younger individuals, with the exception of temporal arteritis and carotidynia.

GENERAL CHARACTERISTICS:
- Shares general characteristics with other deep somatic pain

- Severity of pain may be from mild to excruciating
- The mode of onset is spontaneous
- The pain cannot be provoked
- There is a pulsating or pulsatile component
- Possible association with sensory changes (prodromal, photophobia, phonophobia), nausea, emesis

MANAGEMENTS:
- Rule out dental etiology
- Referral to Oral Medicine or Neurologist or another appropriate medical specialty

TEMPORAL ARTERITIS

Temporal arteritis is a systemic immune, granulomatous condition that affects branches of the carotid artery. This condition may be associated with polymyalgia rheumatica or may arise on its own. Women are affected three times more often than men. The usual age at onset is after the age of 50 years. There appears to be a higher incidence of the condition in northern latitudes. The cause is presumed to be autoimmune. Blindness may occur in one of three untreated patients.

GENERAL CHARACTERISTICS:
- Masticatory muscle pain and fatigue brought on by chewing
- Fever, fatigue, malaise, anorexia, weight loss, and night sweats
- Headache
- Ocular symptoms
- Blurred vision, loss of vision
- Absence of lymphadenopathy
- Scalp tenderness
- Elevated erythrocyte sedimentation rate
- Biopsy confirmation (i.e., giant cells) (*NOTE: a negative biopsy does not preclude therapy*)
- Induration and/or palpation tenderness over the superficial temporal artery
- Jaw claudication

MANAGEMENTS:
- Rule out dental causation
- Rule out/in possibility of referral pain form cervical area
- Referral to Oral Medicine
- Laboratory serum studies (erythrocyte sedimentation rate)
- Referral to Rheumatology and Ophthalmology
- High-dose steroids (to be administered by clinicians experienced in this diagnosis and treatment)

SYMPATHETICALLY MAINTAINED PAIN

Complex Regional Pain Syndrome type I; formerly Reflex Sympathetic Dystrophy

Complex Regional Pain Syndrome type II; formerly Causalgia

The cause of sympathetically maintained pain involves altered regional adrenergic neurotransmission, central nervous system sensitization, neuroplasticity and possible neurogenic inflammation. The symptoms of CRPS I and CRPS II are the same, but the latter has an identifiable peripheral lesion or a history of trauma. CRPS may affect lower or upper limbs and is relatively rare in the head and neck.

GENERAL CHARACTERISTICS:
- Protracted and steady pain
- Mild to severe pain
- Erythema may be present at the site of pain
- Often described as burning
- Poorly localized/diffuse pain
- May be described as phantom pain in an edentulous area
- May begin spontaneously or be brought on by chewing
- May refer to other structures
- May be associated with local tissue atrophy and erythema
- Rule out dental causation; do not treat dentally without a definitive diagnosis
- Hyperpathia
- Allodynia

MANAGEMENTS:
- Rule out dental cause
- Refer to Oral Medicine
- Refer to Anesthesia, Neurology, or other physicians
- Stellate ganglion blockades may assist in the diagnosis and therapy
- Diagnostic phentoalamine systemic adrenergic blockade may be considered.
- At present, therapeutics such as clonidine are experimental

Surgery is inappropriate for this condition.

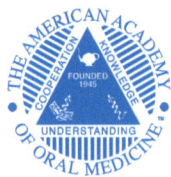

2 Atypical Facial Pain (Persistent Idiopathic Facial Pain)

Persistent pain in the absence of obvious causative factors is common yet is frustrating to providers and patients alike. When it occurs in the facial region, it may be termed atypical facial pain (AFP) (Figure 2–1). A preferable term is persistent idiopathic facial pain (PIFP). It is a form of neuropathic pain and it has been described in many ways. AFP should it occur in the dentoalveolar region has been termed persistent dentoalveolar pain (PDAP). Should it be perceived as pain emanating from a tooth, it may be referred to as atypical odontalgia (AO). Should it occur in an area where a tooth formerly had been, it may be called phantom tooth pain (PTP). The principal mechanism is thought to be neuropathy due to central sensitization, although pain reactions may be conditioned by psychosocial issues. AFP has, in fact, some common features and can usually be separated from such clear-cut entities as trigeminal neuralgia. The etiology of AFP/ PIFP in individual cases is often unknown but may have onset following trauma, treatment, or without any identifiable rationale.

GENERAL CHARACTERISTICS:

- Predominantly women
- 35 to 45 years of age (usually)
- Maxilla greater than mandible (nasolabial fold, marionette line)
- Diffuse pain
- Steady, boring, continuous, deep ache
- Often many previous medical/dental appointments/ procedures
- Does not interfere with sleep
- Pain lasts for varying lengths of time
- Pain of varying intensity
- Florid terms of description (i.e., "Like a knife stuck in my face")
- Usually begins unilaterally but can become bilateral but may have no anatomic distribution
- Worse under stress
- Persisting/recurrent nature of pain
- Temporary remissions (at times after treatment)
- Invasive treatments may worsen the condition

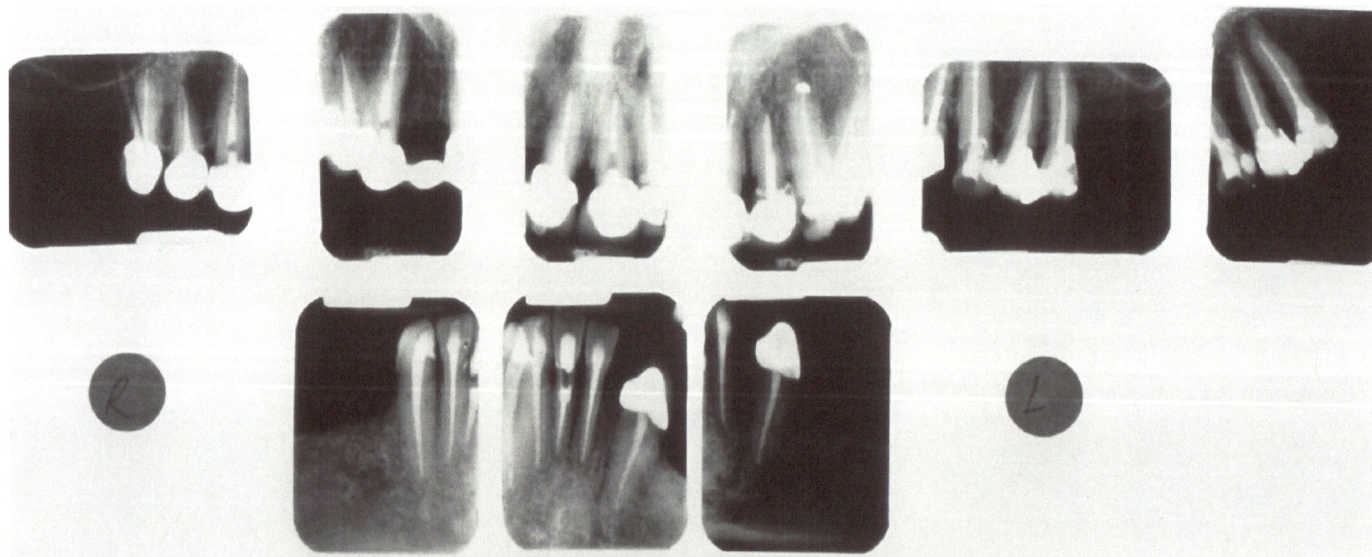

FIGURE 2-1: *Radiographic appearance consistent with atypical facial pain*

Depressive and obsessive behaviors may be observed in some patients and may be either primary or secondary but, in either case, may affect patient symptoms and presentation. Frequently, the patients have seen many practitioners, and often a large number of noninvasive and invasive modalities of treatment have been tried. Many patients are very reluctant to believe that the cause for their pain is not known and will move from practitioner to practitioner insisting that something be done to relieve the problem (termed chronic benign intractable pain syndrome). It is important to recognize that these patients constitute a highly selected sample determined by the severity of the disorder and tenacity in seeking help. The clinician should persist in determining the correct diagnosis to provide effective treatment and not succumb to the patient's desperate demands to initiate invasive procedures, which will usually fail and will often exacerbate the condition. An important, inexpensive diagnostic procedure to consider should be local anesthetic block or infiltration. For example, in a case of suspected AO of tooth #19, if local anesthetic block or osseous infiltration does not eliminate the pain and there are no clinical/radiographic findings, a diagnosis of AO should be entertained. A Technetium-99m Bone Scan of the area may be helpful in some cases to distinguish between an inflammatory versus neuropathic etiology of pain. Consideration of other differential diagnoses, such as carotidynia, complex regional pain syndrome, cancer, central nervous system disease, and myofascial referred pain, is important.

MANAGEMENTS:
- Rule out oral/dental causation
- Rule out neurologic causation
- Refer to Oral Medicine
- Refer to Neurology
- Refer to Psychiatry/Psychology
- Refer to Radiology (for further imaging)

MANAGEMENTS:
The starting point for treatment is a discussion of the diagnosis and ruling out other possible conditions. The discussion should include the nature of the AFP/PIFP, the lack of dangerous physical conditions, and the possibility that the illness may be aggravated by stress. Simple analgesics (e.g., acetaminophen, ibuprofen) may be offered for treatment, but in most cases, the atypical pain patient will already have tried this approach and need further attention. The next step with regard to medications would be to pursue centrally acting medications such as antidepressant, Antiseizure, and anxiolytic therapeutics.5-7 (See tricyclic antidepressant therapy in sections on postherpetic neuralgia and burning mouth syndrome.) Patients may require multidisciplinary management, including psychosocial support, neurology referral, medication support, physical therapy, and possibly counseling.

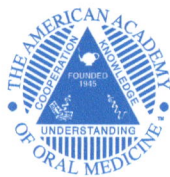

3 Burning Mouth Syndrome/Glossodynia

Burning mouth syndrome (BMS), also known as glossodynia, is an intraoral chronic pain disorder that causes burning discomfort in the absence of oral lesions. Most cases have a spontaneous onset. The most common sites are the anterior two-thirds of the tongue, the anterior hard palate, and the mucosa of the lower lip. Symptoms that frequently accompany BMS include xerostomia (dry mouth), thirst, and dysgeusia (altered taste). Burning often begins by late morning and reaches maximum intensity by evening. The burning is usually continuous and may make falling asleep at night difficult for some patients, although BMS seldom wakes patients during the night. Pain may be reduced with eating, in contrast to pain owing to mucosal lesions, where local stimulation increases pain. Dysgeusia may be present and causes alteration in the ability to taste bitter, sweet and sour compared with control subjects.

Epidemiology
The majority of patients are peri- and post-menopausal females; the gender ratio demonstrates a preponderance of women to men by 3 to 1 or greater. The overall population prevalence is from 0.7 to 2.6%.

GENERAL CHARACTERISTICS:
- Mainly peri- and post-menopausal women
- Women to men ratio, 3 to 1
- Population prevalence 0.7 to 2.6%
- Usually after 40 years of age
- Continuous or intermittent pain
- Burning pain
- Association with xerostomia

MANAGEMENTS:
- Rule out intraoral causation
- Force fluids/xerostomia therapy as necessary
- Rule out oral candidiasis
- Rule out drug reaction (i.e., angiotensin-converting enzyme inhibitors)
- Rule out irritation reaction (i.e., tartar control products)
- Rule out nutritional deficiencies (i.e., iron, folate, vitamin B12, etc.)
- Rule out diabetic neuropathy (i.e., hemoglobin A1c or fasting serum glucose)
- Rule out autoimmune dysfunction (i.e., oral lichen planus)
- Patient education regarding avoiding parafunctional habits
- Evaluate for ill-fitting dentures
- Referral to Oral Medicine

TREATMENT MODALITIES FOR BMS WITH CONCOMITANT XEROSTOMIA
- Increase fluids (water and fruit juices)
- Discontinue or decrease caffeinated beverages, ethanol, and spices
- Discontinue or limit antimuscarinic (drying) drugs (consultation with the patient's physician may be necessary)
- Sialagogue therapy (Referral to Oral Medicine or another appropriate specialty may be necessary. See Treatment below.)
- Palliation: saliva replacements. Consider over-the-counter products, such as artificial saliva, dry-mouth chewing gum, nonalcoholic mouthwash (i.e., Biotin products, Oral Balance Dry Mouth Moisturizing Gel, Oasis Mouth Spray).

> **Rx**: Pilocarpine hydrochloride (Salagen) 5 mg tablets*
> Disp: 100 tablets
> Sig: Take 1 tablet tid or qid times daily

* Sweating and flushing are the most common side effects. Contraindicated in patients with uncontrolled asthma.

> **Rx**: Cevimeline (Evoxac) 30 mg tablets*
> Disp: 100 tablets
> Sig: Take 1 tablet tid daily

* Contraindicated in patients with uncontrolled asthma and narrow-angle glaucoma.

TREATMENT MODALITIES FOR SYMPTOMS OF BURNING

- Blood studies to rule out nutritional deficiency (i.e., especially CBC, Fe++, vitamin B12 [methylmalonic acid], folic acid, and Zn++) and replacement as necessary. (Referral to Oral Medicine or a physician may be necessary.)
- Rule out oral vesiculoerosive disease (i.e., lichen planus) oral candidiasis
- Rule out diabetic neuropathy
- Trial hormonal replacement therapy if premenopausal (refer to physician)
- Autoimmune serum studies (i.e., erythrocyte sedimentation rate, antinuclear factor, Sjögren's syndrome antigens A and B, rheumatoid factor, and complement levels)
- Rule in or rule out material, drug, and food allergy and/or intolerance as necessary
- Benzodiazepine (clonazepam), tricyclic antidepressant (TCA) (low dose), capsaicin, and gabapentin therapies. (It is suggested that patients be referred to Oral Medicine or other appropriate specialists for these therapies.)

Clonazepam Therapy:

> **Rx**: Clonazepam 1 mg tablets*
> Disp: 100 tablets
> Sig: Take ½ to 1 tablet for 3 min and spit out. In the am, let ½ to 1 tablet melt in mouth for 3 min and spit out. In the pm, let ½ to 1 tablet melt in mouth for 3 min and spit out. At bedtime, let ½ to 1 tablet melt in mouth for 3 min and spit out. (Some studies have assessed local application, others systemic dosing)

* As clonazepam may alter concentration and coordination, do not drive a car or operate machinery until reasonably capable. It may take several days to adjust to the medication before the patient is able to drive after the initiation of therapy. It may take several weeks before the beneficial effects of the medication are manifested.

Low-Dose TCA Therapy:

> **Rx**: Amitriptyline 10 or 25 mg tablets
> Disp: 40 tablets
> Sig: Take 1 tablet hs.

> **Rx**: Nortriptyline 10 or 25 mg tablets
> Disp: 40 tablets
> Sig: Take 1 tablet hs.

The dose can be increased slowly, titrated up to effect or side effect on a gradual basis. After 1 week (if there is no perceived benefit), increase the dosage by one 25 mg tablet (or 10 mg tablet) and 4 weeks later (if there is still no perceived benefit) by one more 25 mg tablet (up to 75 mg per day) depending on the patient's tolerance of the medication. TCAs may need 2 to 3 weeks before they become effective in relieving pain. TCAs are known to cause some drowsiness initially or on increasing the dosage regimen. Further, they are known to cause xerostomia and have other known side effects. After continued pain relief, the dosage should be titrated down and discontinued. Other TCAs, such as doxepin and desipramine, are also effective in the treatment of chronic pain.

NOTE: **Spontaneous remission and partial spontaneous remission may occur within 6 or 7 years after onset in more than half of patients with chronic oral burning. Remission may be preceded by a change in the pattern of burning from constant to episodic.**

> **Rx**: Capsaicin (Zostrix crm) 0.025%*
> Disp: 1 tube
> Sig: Apply a small dab to affected area tid or qid.

*Substance P is a mediator of pain. It is associated with the transmission of pain with an aching and burning quality. Capsaicin is a depleter of substance P and the active component of red chili peppers. Capsaicin is applied to burning tissues to down regulate nociception. Capsaicin is applied to the patient's painful oral mucosa according to the individual's tolerance. Caution patient about the initial application might cause C-fiber activation and pain; however, repeated application causes gradual desensitization.

SUMMARY

BMS remains relatively unexplored and unexplained in regard to many aspects of etiology, diagnosis, and therapy. The diagnosis of BMS is a diagnosis of exclusion of other differential diagnoses. Therapeutic outcomes are usually successful. The clinician is directed to evaluate the published relevant data to maximize the success of treatment.

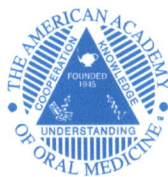

4 Temporomandibular Disorders: Myogenous and Arthrogenous Conditions

Temporomandibular disorders (TMDs) are a major source of face, head, and neck pain. They may be separated into arthrogenous and myogenous categories, and there are several subcategories within each. A diagnostic system based on physical factors (Axis I) and psychological factors (Axis II) was modified in 2014. These are called the Diagnostic Criteria for Temporomandibular Disorders (DC/TMD). On the clinical level, a system based on differential diagnosis and description of signs and symptoms is the most widely used. These disorders have been a source of considerable controversy in the dental community, based on different concepts about diagnosis, etiology, and therapy. Nevertheless, the scientific clinical communities responsible for the diagnosis and treatment of these conditions have reached a high level of agreement about how TMD patients should be managed, especially with regard to the early phases of these conditions. This section emphasizes the currently accepted conservative (reversible) treatment strategies that have been shown to be effective in over 75 to 80% of primary TMD patients. Unfortunately, there is no consensus about how treatment-resistant and other chronic TMD patients should be managed, although it is evident that management approaches consistent with other chronic pain states are necessary.

When clinicians first encounter any type of orofacial pain, including TMD, their main efforts should be directed to rule out odontogenic conditions and at providing successful early treatment, which in itself is often the best way to avoid the development of chronicity.

Successful early treatment programs should offer the following benefits to TMD patients:

1. A proper scientific explanation about the nature and prognosis of their disorder
2. Relief from pain throughout the treatment period to enhance recovery
3. Self-management strategies and procedures for home care
4. When indicated, oral appliances to decrease excessive parafunctional oral activity and joint loading
5. Over-the-counter analgesics as needed
6. After completion of treatment, instructions for avoidance and self-management of future recurrences

The question of why some TMD/myofascial pain disorder (MPD) patients respond to initial therapies and others do not is not clearly understood. Studies have attempted to find possible physical or psychological variables that might account for these different outcomes. While no consistent predictors of treatment outcome have been found, emerging data shows that TMD patients who present with other comorbid functional pain disorders such as fibromyalgia, irritable bowel syndrome and chronic headache, tend to be more difficult to treat. Alterations in central pain processing networks are the proposed pathophysiology. Although the majority of patients do improve (regression to the mean) with time, another factor that complicates the management of chronic TMD/MPD cases is the lack of a clear understanding about the etiology of these conditions. However, because many of the past etiologic theories in the TMD/MPD field are based on mechanistic concepts of craniomandibular misalignment, improper vertical dimension, occlusal disharmonies, dentoalveolar discrepancies, and so on, we frequently see nonresponding TMD patients being treated with increasingly aggressive dental therapies. Likewise, the failure to understand why some TMD patients do not get better often leads to inappropriate proposals for surgical interventions inside the temporomandibular joint (TMJ). These illogical thinking processes may lead to horrific outcomes for chronic TMD patients because they may result in treatment resistant combinations of chronic pain and irreversible post dental or postsurgical problems.

Two recent papers have dealt with this subject of irreversible treatments for TMD from an ethical standpoint and from a medical necessity viewpoint. Reid and Greene laid out an ethical framework for dental and medical professionals to consider when recommending treatments for various types of TMD patients. While a small number of very specific conditions may require extensive dental or surgical solutions, the evidence is very strong to support the routine use of conservative and reversible modalities for most patients. Therefore, suggesting a need for more aggressive treatments (and of course actually carrying out those treatments) can be described as a breach of professional ethics. In the paper by Greene and Obrez, a framework for evaluating the medical necessity of jaw repositioning was proposed, and current treatments for TMD problems were discussed within that framework. Their conclusion was that the various procedures proposed by advocates of such therapies generally could not meet the test of medical necessity, and therefore they should be regarded as inappropriate treatments.

MYOGENOUS TMDS

There are several types of myogenous TMDs, but the most common ones seem to be myalgia and myofascial pain and dysfunction, which is similar to such problems elsewhere in the body. The current understanding of masticatory myalgia is that it is a multifactorial condition with several contributing factors that vary in importance from one patient to another. This concept is a topic of ongoing research, and clinicians who treat TMD/MPD must keep current by reading recent literature. The major factors currently believed to play an important role in the etiology of muscle pain include the following:

Trauma. Direct trauma to the mandible can stretch and tear the masticatory muscles and lead to muscle spasm and pain. Indirect trauma, such as flexion extension injuries (whiplash), may also be a cause of masticatory myogenous pain and dysfunction in some cases, but most cases of whiplash do not automatically lead to the development of pain in the masticatory muscles.

Parafunctional Habits. Nocturnal bruxism and daytime clenching of the teeth are believed to be an important factor or cofactor in myalgia, and treatment directed toward decreasing these habits is an important component of therapy. Muscle fatigue is an often underappreciated source of pain in TMD. Excess muscle activity leads to lactate, ATP, and pH changes which sensitive group III and IV muscle afferents via TRPV1, P2X and ASIC3 receptors respectively. Since masticatory muscles are governed

by the trigeminal nerve, these signals bombard the subnucleus caudalis of the trigeminal brainstem nuclei; an area that receives nociceptive input from cranial nerves V, VII, IX and X as well as cervical nerves as caudal as C4.

Psychosocial Factors. Anxiety and depression appear to play an important role in initiating and perpetuating myofascial pain by increasing both muscular hyperactivity and the patient's reaction to pain. Some clinicians argue that psychological disturbance, when present, is mainly related to (1) selection factors (a very common problem) and (2) demonstrable psychological consequences of chronic pain. Clinicians who do not consider the psychological aspects of myalgia will have more difficulty in successfully managing patients with this condition, especially patients with symptoms resistant to conservative, noninvasive or reversible methods of therapy.

Occlusion. A sudden change in the occlusal condition with a new restoration may recruit new muscle engrams that lead to muscle fatigue and pain. Outside that setting, occlusal abnormalities are no longer believed to be the major cause of myalgia; they may be a contributing factor in certain subsets of patients when introduced during dental treatment. Research to date leads to the conclusion that initial therapy should not be directed toward permanent changes in the occlusion.

Systemic disorders not localized to the jaws, which may play a role in causing symptoms of masticatory muscle pain, include fibromyalgia, polymyalgia rheumatica, somatization disorders, and chronic fatigue syndrome.

MANAGEMENT OF MYALGIA AND MYOFASCIAL PAIN

Conservative Management Strategies

Management of muscular pain and dysfunction should begin with a discussion of the condition with the patient. (The assumption is made that dental causes, that is, pericoronitis and dental abscesses, have been ruled out.) It is essential to rule out (or in) other diagnoses, such as infection and neoplasm, to ensure that more serious diagnoses are not overlooked. Several facts need to be presented to educate the patient about the nature of this muscular condition. Myofascial pain and dysfunction may be self-limiting. It is possible for resolution to occur within a reasonable period of time regardless of which treatment modalities are employed. However, some patients will not respond favorably to initial therapies, so clinicians should be aware of perpetuating factors that may be impediments to successful treatment.

Common perpetuating factors include the following:

- Mechanical stresses: skeletal asymmetry, poor posture, and abuse of muscles
- Allergies: inhalant, ingested, contact
- Chronic inflammatory disorders: chronic infection, connective tissue diseases
- Metabolic and endocrine factors: hypothyroidism, hyperuricemia, hypoglycemia
- Psychological factors: depression, anxiety

Depression is a common result of chronic pain and acts as a perpetuating factor. There is no scientific evidence that depression is a primary etiologic factor in chronic pain, nor is it surprising that persistent pain is often accompanied by anxiety, especially prior to diagnosis. Sleep may be impacted by chronic pain. Both depression and anxiety may regress with successful pain management. Therefore, it is often necessary to direct resources to the appropriate management of pain, sleep dysfunction, depression or anxiety as soon as possible.

We suggest prompt **noninvasive reversible therapy** for most masticatory myalgia and myofascial pain. Such therapy includes a **soft diet, moist heat, and medications**. When pain is severe and acute, application of cold will significantly contribute to pain reduction. Medications include the judicious use of analgesics (usually nonsteroidal anti-inflammatory drugs [NSAIDs]), muscle relaxants, and adjuvant analgesics such as tricyclic antidepressants (TCAs) and anticonvulsants. Nonaggressive therapy can be helpful and economical. Moist heat modalities (hot water bottles, warm to hot packs, and electric heating pads) should be used for approximately one half-hour and at least one half-hour of rest before the next initiation of moist heat therapy. With respect to traumatic injury, time and the capacity of the body's inherent ability to heal are the greatest clinical resources. Therefore, the main treatment objective is to allow the patient to be comfortable while healing continues.

Habit Reversal Therapy

The patient will need to be instructed to find positions of rest for the jaw, tongue and head. The patient should choose a visual or auditory reminder within their work and home space in order to prompt them to check themselves to make sure 1) Teeth are slightly apart. 2) Tongue lays in the floor of the mouth. Instruct patient to puff air gently through lips and then rest their face. This should place their teeth slightly apart and tongue in a neutral position. 3) Neutral head posture.

Exercise

Passive, non-painful stretch exercises for the muscles of mastication may prove helpful. Exercises should not be used past the point where they initiate pain. The objective of stretching exercise is to regain muscle length and coordination. TMD self-care and home-care instructions with patient education should be considered.

Vapocoolant Spray and Stretch

Spray and stretch is a noninvasive technique for both diagnosis and therapy of myofascial pain and can be readily accomplished as an office procedure. Palpation of the involved muscles may locate tender points or taut muscle fiber bands (also referred to as trigger points) in a specific area of muscle. Once this tender point is located and identified in a specific muscle, knowledge of muscle physiology and anatomy is needed to stretch the muscle to its full physiologic length after spraying. The spray acts as a sensory confounder, which allows passive stretch. The stretch itself is thought to be the therapeutic action.

The general procedure is as follows:

- Locate the tender point and identify the muscle.
- Direct the stream of liquid at a 45° angle to the skin surface overlying the muscle.
- Using overlapping strokes parallel to the muscle fibers, spray the entire muscle length in the direction of pain referral, culminating at the pain reference site.
- Stretch the muscle passively to its full physiologic length but short of the point of producing pain.
- After completing spray and stretch, apply moist heat over the area for a few minutes.
- Repeat above up to three times.
- Have the patient perform range of motion exercises to actively stretch the muscle and allow measurement or estimation of progress.

Care must be taken not to frost the skin or chill the underlying muscle excessively and especially not to endanger the eye. The most acceptable spray agent currently available is Fluori-Methane, but a more "environment-friendly" coolant is under development.

An alternative to Fluori-Methane can be purchased OTC by patient (Max-Freeze with a roll-on Formula) for at home using above technique. For a detailed description of the procedure for each muscle, the reader is referred to the books by Simons and Travell.

Stretch without Spray (Lewit Technique Modified by Simons)

This post-isometric muscle relaxation technique is effective in treating myofascial pain and can be taught to the patient to complement or supplement an exercise program. The directions below are for the patient:

1. While in a well-supported, relaxed position, stretch the involved muscle in a gentle, non-painful manner.
2. Holding this position, apply gentle counter pressure with a hand and contract the muscle for about 3 seconds. Then release and relax the muscle completely.
3. Inhale deeply and while exhaling allow the muscle to stretch, taking up all of the slack that develops. Stop stretching after exhaling. Do not stretch to the point where it becomes painful.
4. Slowly and gently move the muscle actively through a complete range of motion three times.
5. Repeat if needed. Warm the muscle if resistance is encountered.

For muscle trigger points that persist, injection with local anesthetics without a vasoconstrictor and botulinum toxin (Botox) injections may be considered.

Trigger point injections

The presence of myofascial trigger points (knots, taut bands) can perpetuate myogenous TMD conditions. Classically, a myofascial trigger point will refer pain to a site remote to the area of palpation. The masseter, trapezius and sternocleidomastoid can all refer pain to the TMJ area. Injecting the trigger point with approximately 0.5 mL of mepivacaine or lidocaine without vasoconstrictor can break up actin-myosin kinks within muscle. Avoid bupivacaine as it can be myotoxic.

Electrotherapeutic Management of Myofascial Pain

Electrical modalities include transcutaneous electric nerve stimulation (TENS), iontophoresis, and high-voltage stimulation. Although these modalities may be used individually, they are employed most often in combination with other forms of myofascial pain treatment. Used in this context, electric modalities may enhance patient comfort and reduce treatment time. Although electrotherapeutic modalities are well established for trunk and extremity pain, their use in the head and neck region is not as well established. They should be used only by clinicians with training in electrotherapeutic modalities.

Transcutaneous Electric Nerve Stimulation:

TENS decreases pain by blocking ascending sensory input ("closing the gate") and by stimulating release of endogenous opiates such as endorphins.

Critical elements of effective TENS are
- Proper electrode placement to cover or bracket trigger points
- Optimal setting: intensity, rate, width, and modulation
- Patient compliance with recommended regimen

Generally, TENS should be used 22 to 24 hours daily for the first 3 days and then tapered to 15 to 18 hours daily for the next several weeks. Improvement and lead placement need to be monitored, and the time of use should be reduced gradually until the patient is asymptomatic. TENS units may be initiated through a referral to physical therapy. For chronic use, the patient may desire to buy a unit after a month's trial.

Iontophoresis

Iontophoresis is a method that uses low-amperage direct current to enhance tissue penetration of ionized drugs. It is based on the law of physics that like charges repel and opposites attract. A positively charged medication such as lidocaine hydrochloride, when placed under a positive electrode, will therefore be driven away from the electrode and into the tissue. The usual depth of penetration is 1 to 2 cm, although traces of drug can be found in deeper tissues. If a corticosteroid is added to the drug delivery electrode, the charge is changed to negative and the process is repeated.

A distinct advantage to iontophoresis is the minimal systemic absorption of drugs and a consequent lack of adverse side effects. The dosage of delivered drug is measured in milliamps per minute. However, several studies have questioned the efficacy of this modality for treating masticatory myofascial pain; therefore, its value is not firmly established.

High-Voltage Stimulation

High-voltage stimulation is an electrotherapeutic modality for muscular disorders that employs a monophasic twin-peak wave of high-voltage current and at the same time produces a very low- average current. Treatment is comfortable and safe for the patient. When combined with stretch and spray treatment, moist heat application, and a muscle-lengthening exercise program; this therapy can be effective and efficient. High-voltage stimulation therapy is available through physical therapy referral.

TABLE 4–1: INDICATIONS FOR THE USE OF ORAL APPLIANCES	
Diagnosis or Signs of Symptoms	*Indications*
Masticatory myalgia	Myalgia resulting from heavy bruxism while awake or sleeping
TMJ arthralgia	Unilateral or bilateral trauma to TMJ soft tissues, possibly from bruxism and/or with a history of polyjoint arthritis
Atypical facial pain/atypical odontalgia/PFPUE	Chronic tooth pain with no evidence of pulpal infection or heavy bruxism
TMJ dysfunction	Painful clicking, episodes of locking, heavy bruxism
Temporary occlusion	Pain in the presence of unstable occlusion owing to tooth loss, supereruption, open bites. If this is not linked to occlusal reconstruction or orthodontic treatment, the patient may be doomed to long-term splint wear.
Bruxism, cracked, chipped, or worn teeth	To protect teeth from heavy bruxism, pain upon awakening
Frequent headaches	Headache history that has not responded to medical management; heavy bruxism with fatigue and inflammation of masticatory muscles
PFPUE = persistent facial pain of unknown etiology; TMJ = temporomandibular joint Adapted from Clark and Minakuchi.	

TABLE 4–2: TYPES OF SPLINTS	
Full Occlusal Night Guard, Stabilization Splint, etc.	*Partial-Coverage Splint, Flat Plane*
Maxillary: relatively easy to adjust (Figure 4-1)	Maxillary anterior: very comfortable, minimized clenching
Mandibular: difficult to adjust anterior relationships; may be annoying to tongue but better esthetics	Maxillary or mandibular bilateral posterior Anterior repositioning appliance (maxillary or mandibular)

OCCLUSAL APPLIANCES, SPLINTS, AND ORTHOTICS IN THE TREATMENT OF CHRONIC OROFACIAL PAIN

Oral appliances are presently viewed as a reasonable adjunctive therapy for some oral pain TMD patients. These oral appliances are often referred to as splints, night guards, or orthotic device. A number of recent studies have cast doubt on the value of splint therapy compared with other therapies as the preferable predictable modality of choice. One group of investigators reported equal success between myofascial pain patients treated with placebo and full-coverage splints. Another group of investigators found no difference between medical management, soft splints, and hard splints, whereas a third group of investigators found no difference in patient improvement comparing stabilizing splints with non-occluding splints.

It is important for the clinician to follow documented indications for the use of an oral appliance (Table 4-1). Treatment decisions should be based on evidence determined from the patient's history and clinical examination. It is important that a treatment plan using the splint be developed and followed at the initiation of therapy.

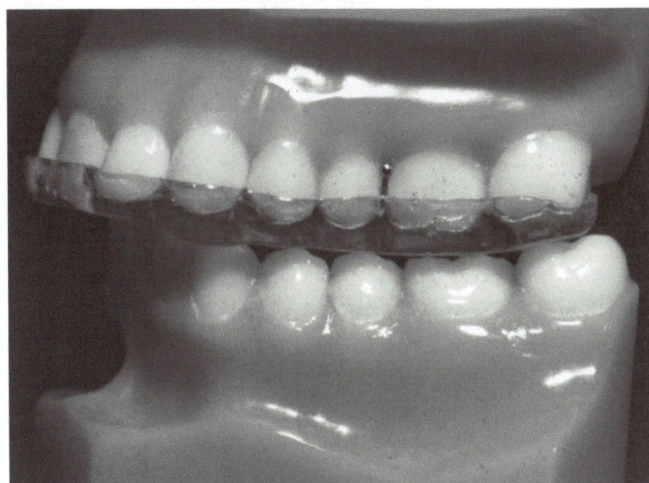

FIGURE 4-1: *Full-coverage occlusal maxillary splint.*

Splints require proper fitting and adjustment. Splints should not cause pain, and splint use should not result in a changed occlusion. Splints are not intended to permanently "recapture" disks or to reposition mandibles. Repositioning of the mandible increases the likelihood that the occlusion will change. Recapturing the disk and repositioning the mandible is viable only with respect to either orthodontic or prosthodontic therapeutic modalities. Patients should be given clear instructions, and regular patient follow-up is highly advised. Conditions listed in Table 4-1 currently advised and indicated for the use of splint therapy.

PATIENT INSTRUCTIONS

- Wear the splint every night when sleeping.
- Wear the splint during the day if experiencing pain.
- Do not wear the splint 24 hours a day.
- Wearing the splint continuously may provoke irreversible problematic changes in the occlusion.
- Do not eat with the splint.

IMPORTANT CLINICIAN INSTRUCTIONS

- The splint should be checked with articulating paper at each patient visit and any wear facets in the acrylic should be flattened to allow opposing teeth to slide easily across the occlusal surface Consider using upper and lower occlusal hard acrylic splints for patients who consistently create deep grooves in the stent during nocturnal bruxism.
- Patients should be scheduled for an initial follow-up and for regular follow-up evaluations.
- If there is pain reduction and the splint is comfortable, these may indicate that the patient is ready to reduce or stop splint wear.
- Patient should stop wearing appliance and return to dentist for an evaluation if pain intensity increased or and parts of appliance fractured.

PHARMACOTHERAPEUTICS

Analgesics

NSAIDs are useful in the management of chronic pain, although controlled studies in the treatment of TMD have not demonstrated efficacy. This class of drugs includes aspirin and aspirin-like drugs. NSAIDs can produce pseudo-allergic reactions in sensitive individuals and must be avoided in individuals with such a history. NSAID therapy has the potential to cause stomach ulcers or increase the severity of gastric ulcerative conditions. Drinking a tall glass of warm water with any medication and taking the medication after food decrease the potential for gastrointestinal distress and help the medication dissolve. Sensitive individuals may demonstrate capillary fragility or bruising with NSAID use. Further, some patients may experience clotting difficulties. Centrally acting analgesics such as acetaminophen lack anti- inflammatory action and therefore may not be as useful as NSAIDs, but in patients with NSAID sensitivity or intolerance, acetaminophen may

be the best available choice. Non-acetylated salicylates are another fallback analgesic drug group for NSAID-allergic or -intolerant patients. Cyclooxygenase II inhibitors, such as celecoxib, are currently on the market for the treatment of arthritis. This class of drugs appears to have excellent analgesic attributes, but also this class of drugs has the potential for increasing cardiac risks and presently does not have an established record in the treatment of orofacial pain. Narcotic analgesics should be avoided in the treatment of chronic pain in most cases. In general, narcotics may be addictive and are a poor choice for long term therapies. For many chronic pain patients, the controlled withdrawal of narcotics and sedatives is a necessary step in treatment. However, in the long-term treatment of intractable pain (i.e., for cancer patients), narcotic analgesics are often a valuable aid (see Chapter 6, "Cancer and Chronic Orofacial Pain"). Further, chronic pain may manifest at times as a severe acute pain episode that may require acutely administered narcotic analgesics. Narcotic analgesics in the treatment of severe pain have only a very limited potential for addiction.

Examples of NSAID Prescriptions for Facial Pain Conditions:

> **Rx**: Aspirin (OTC) 325 mg tablets
> Disp: 500 tablets
> Sig: Take 3 tablets qid pc and hs for at least 2 wk.

> **Rx**: Ibuprofen (OTC) 200 mg tablets
> Disp: 500 tablets
> Sig: Take 3 tablets qid for at least 2 wk pc and hs.

> **Rx**: Naproxen 500 mg tablets
> Disp: 100 tablets
> Sig: Take 1 tablet bid for at least 2 wk pc and hs.

Other NSAIDs, such as flurbiprofen, phenylbutazone, sulindac, diflunisal, piroxicam, indomethacin, meclofenamate, fenoprofen, mefenamic acid, tolmetin, and diclofenac, may be used depending on the patient's medical status and the chronicity of the pain.

Example of Acetaminophen Prescription

> **Rx**: Acetaminophen (OTC) 325 mg
> Disp: 500 tablets
> Sig: Take 2 tablets qid prn.

An Example of Nonacetylated Salicylates

> **Rx**: Disalcid 750 mg tablets
> Disp: 100 tablets
> Sig: Take 2 tablets bid prn.

Anticonvulsants

Carbamazepine, phenytoin, and baclofen are used in the treatment of facial neuralgia such as trigeminal neuralgia. These drugs are difficult to titrate and have several problematic side effects. Phenytoin has a half-life of approximately 1 month, which complicates maintaining the serum level within the therapeutic window. Carbamazepine is known for liver toxicity and blood dyscrasias. Therefore, liver function blood studies are necessary at regular intervals. Allergic hypersensitivity is another concern with these drugs. These drugs may induce liver enzymes, which further complicates patient management. Gabapentin is another potential therapeutic; however, controlled studies regarding the efficacy of gabapentin in the treatment of chronic orofacial pain have not been completed at this time. Therefore, anticonvulsants should be used only by clinicians educated in the therapeutic management of anticonvulsant pharmacotherapeutics for pain control.

Muscle Relaxants

These drugs are helpful as an adjunct when combined with another muscle therapy (e.g., moist heat, splint therapy). Benzodiazepines such as diazepam (Valium) have limited efficacy. Benzodiazepines have an addictive potential, which can be a significant liability in the treatment of chronic pain. When used at all, benzodiazepines should be limited to a particular duration of time (although clonazepam therapy in the treatment of burning mouth syndrome has shown efficacy in clinical trials). Muscle relaxers available include cyclobenzaprine (Flexeril), methocarbamol (Robaxin), tizanidine (Zanaflex), metaxalone (Skelaxin), chlorzoxazone (Parafon forte), carisoprodol (Soma) and baclofen (Lioresal). As a class they are generally sedating so they are best used at bedtime. Methocarbamol is less sedating and is generally tolerated even during the day. Tizanidine may be considered with patients in whom stress aggravates their pain. If muscle spasticity is present, baclofen may be an option.

Example of Muscle Relaxant Prescriptions:

> **Rx**: Cyclobenzaprine 5 or 10 mg tablets
> Disp: 21 tablets
> Sig: Take 1 tablet hs. daily for 3 weeks

> **Rx**: Methocarbamol 500 mg tablets
> Disp: 84 or 168 tablets
> Sig: Take 1–2 tablets tid to qid daily for 3 weeks

> **Rx**: Tizanidine 2 mg tablets
> Disp: 21 tablets
> Sig: Take 1 tablet hs. for 3 weeks

Drowsiness is a possible side effect; therefore, patients should be cautioned concerning driving.

Tricyclic Antidepressants

Some TCAs have been scientifically proved to be effective in the treatment of chronic orofacial pain. These drugs (i.e., amitriptyline, desipramine, doxepin, nortriptyline, etc.) alleviate many chronic pain conditions through their analgesic effects rather than their antidepressant benefits. (See the section on postherpetic neuralgia or burning mouth syndrome for further information.)

TMJ ARTICULAR DISORDERS

Whereas myofascial pain is responsible for the majority of chronic orofacial musculoskeletal pain, articular disorders of the TMJ are a less common cause of chronic orofacial pain. TMJ articular disorders may be classified in various ways based on anatomic structures that are affected, inflammatory versus non-inflammatory components present, or another presumed etiology. As with TMDs in general, no classification system has gained full acceptance as an ideal system.

In addition, many classes of TMJ articular disorders have significant overlap with other articular disorders, thus further hindering a generally accepted classification system. For the purposes of this monograph, the classification will be based on anatomic structures that are affected. These categories include:

- Disorders affecting the *articular disc*
- Disorders affecting the *condylar head* or *glenoid fossa*

In this section, we list particular disorders and review present etiologic theories. It is important to review validity and reliability of these conditions. Please see study by Schiffman et al. listed in reference section.

Disorders of the Articular Disk-Disk Derangement (and Adhesions)

ETIOLOGY:

Displacement with and without reduction of the articular disk (stretched, torn, or perforated disk) can result from various factors (see below):

- Trauma (macrotrauma): results in capsulitis/synovitis and can alter disk dynamics. This results from direct injury to the jaw, including condylar fracture, flexion/extension injury (whiplash) to the mandible, or prolonged hyperextension of the mandible during eating or dental treatment.
- Microtrauma: prolonged joint loading from parafunction or resting teeth together over many years may exceed the adaptive capacity of the dense, fibrous connective of the TMJ articular disc and the fibrocartilage linings of the mandibular condyle and glenoid fossa. With time, morphologic changes to these structures may lead to condylar flattening and osteophyte formation. In the case of the disc, structural changes lead to anteromedial disc displacements due to the orientation and pull of the lateral pterygoid muscle in that direction. This process is an asymptomatic one in most people. One in three people have a disc displacement of one kind or another.
- Joint laxity/joint hypermobility: inherited predisposition studies have confirmed a correlation between generalized joint laxity and predisposition to TMJ disk displacement alone or in combination with condylar subluxation (patient is able to reduce the joint)/luxation (dentist manipulates and reduces joint).

CLINICAL FINDINGS

TABLE 4–3: DISC DISPLACEMENT WITH REDUCTION, DISC DISPLACEMENT WITHOUT REDUCTION (CLOSED LOCK)	
Reciprocal Clicking	*Severely Restricted Jaw Movement*
Symptomatic or asymptomatic	May be associated with pain in preauricular area
Little or no movement, restriction associated with deviation at time of click	Less painful jaw deflection to affected side
Radiographs usually normal; best visualized with magnetic resonance imaging	

MANAGEMENTS:

- No treatment is necessary for asymptomatic clicks.
- For an inflammatory pain component, NSAID therapy may be recommended.
- Consider oral appliance therapy.
- When there is persistent joint inflammation and/or associated fibrosis/adhesions, refer to appropriate clinical resources for intra-articular steroid injection or arthrocentesis (i.e., lysis and lavage—Oral and Maxillofacial Surgery).

Disorders Affecting the Condylar Head/Fossa/Joint Capsule Arthritides

(See Table 4 – 4, next page)

MANAGEMENTS: (See Table 4–5, next page)
Other examples of arthritis within the temporomandibular complex include septic, psoriatic, and gouty joints. These entities are rare and require referral to appropriate specialists.

Congenital Abnormalities or Developmental Defects

GENERAL CHARACTERISTICS:

- Includes patients with aplasia (agenesis), hypoplasia, hyperplasia, neoplasia of the condyle
- Primarily causes cosmetic or functional problems rarely associated with orofacial pain unless seen with neoplasia; movement and deviation of the jaw are to the affected side
- Differential diagnosis includes all disorders of the TMJ, including neoplasm, trauma, inflammatory arthritis, and significant bone remodeling due to non-inflammatory conditions.

MANAGEMENTS: Refer the patient to Oral Medicine/Oral and Maxillofacial Surgery.

Temporomandibular Derangements of Joint

GENERAL CHARACTERISTICS:

- Usually occurs in patients with predisposition to laxity, that is, hypermobile joints
- May result from trauma
- Occurs most often when the condylar head moves anterior to articular eminence
- Acute inability to close mouth fully (Closed Locked)
- Acute inability to close at all with mouth wide open (Open Locked)
- Dislocation with severe pain, which recedes with time
- Radiograph will confirm the condyle past the eminence

Disorders Affecting the Condylar Head/Fossa/Joint Capsule Arthritides (Table 4 – 4)

TABLE 4–4: TYPES OF ARTHRITIS	
Osteoarthritis/Degenerative Joint	*Rheumatoid Arthritis Disease*
Primarily a non-inflammatory degeneration of the articular surface of the joint leading to bone remodeling	A systemic inflammatory process that can lead to vasculitis of the synovial membrane of the TMJ, leading to progressive deterioration of bone
May result from an imbalance between predominantly chondrocyte controlled processes that result in a progressive degeneration of the articular surface	May involve multiple joints in a patient
May be the result of excessive joint loading; an identifiable initiating factor has not been discovered	May affect both older and younger (i.e., juvenile rheumatoid arthritis) age groups
Most common internal derangement in patients over 50 yr. old	Radiographs show bone deterioration
Can be associated with a secondary inflammation of synovium (often associated with micro/macro trauma)	May lead to open bite if bilateral deterioration occurs
Sometimes no symptomatology	Hematologic parameters may yield positive rheumatoid factor
Can be associated with pain	Patient may have crepitus during jaw during function movement
Patient may have pointed tenderness in the joint	Pain at rest in the preauricular area
Radiographic evidence of structural bony change and joint space narrowing or osteophytes	Pain on palpation of preauricular area
Secondary findings may occur including limited range of motion, crepitus, deviation of mandible on opening noted to affected side	Other oral or systemic autoimmune manifestations (i.e., Sjögren's syndrome, Reiter syndrome)

TABLE 4–5: ARTHRITIS MANAGEMENT	
Osteoarthritis	*Rheumatoid Arthritis*
Must rule out capsulitis without bony changes, other inflammatory polyarthritides, and neoplasia	Must differentiate from osteoarthritis, capsulitis, other inflammatory arthritides, ear infection, and neoplasia
Conservative medical management or refer to Oral Medicine	Refer to Oral Medicine
Refer to Internal Medicine/Rheumatology	Refer to Internal Medicine/Rheumatology

- Can be unilateral or bilateral and momentary (subluxation) or long lasting (luxation)
- Differential diagnosis includes fractured condyle

MANAGEMENTS: Refer the patient to Oral Medicine/Oral and Maxillofacial Surgery.

Inflammatory Capsulitis/Synovitis
GENERAL CHARACTERISTICS:
- Usually related to or followed by a traumatic event
- Localized pain with function in the preauricular area or external auditory meatus

- Limitation of opening secondary to pain, less than 40 mm inter-incisal opening
- The patient may note a hyperocclusion
- Within the differential diagnosis, it is necessary to rule out osteoarthritis, disk disorder, inflammatory arthritides, ear infection, and neoplasia

MANAGEMENTS: Refer to the section on treatment for myofascial pains.

Ankylosis

GENERAL CHARACTERISTICS:

- A true fusion (soft tissue or bony) of the condylar head to the glenoid fossa
- The condition is usually related to trauma or extended joint immobilization
- Patient might have had a history of joint adhesions
- Limited range of motion on opening
- The jaw moves to the affected side
- The condition may not be painful if chronic
- Radiographs reveal absence of condylar movement with obliteration of joint space if the bones are fused
- Within the differential diagnosis, it is necessary to rule out disc dislocation without reduction, muscle contracture.

MANAGEMENTS: Consider consultation with Oral and Maxillofacial Surgery.

Neoplasm of the Jaw Joint Tissue

GENERAL CHARACTERISTICS:

- Various neoplasms of malignant or benign etiology can involve the temporomandibular complex
- The most common benign neoplasm of the temporomandibular complex is the Osteochondroma. Synovial chondromatosis, which is secondary to an abnormal production of cartilaginous material owing to a metaplasia of the synovium, typically affects large joints and is rare in the TMJ. But when present, produces symptoms of pain and decreased range of motion of the jaw. See below CBCT and 3D illustrated image of an Osteochondroma in head of left condyle (arrows)
- Malignant neoplasms of the temporomandibular complex can emanate from local tissue, that is, osteosarcoma/chondrosarcoma, or from a distant malignant disease
- Clinical findings include pain, swelling, capsulitis, limited jaw movement, pathologic fracture, and opening to the affected side
- Radiographs may show bone deterioration; magnetic resonance imaging in synovial chondromatosis may show "joint mice" (small cartilaginous material in joint capsule)
- Within the differential diagnosis, it is necessary to rule out all other joint pathologies/conditions, disc disorders, non-inflammatory and inflammatory arthritis, and trauma

MANAGEMENTS: Refer the patient to appropriate clinical resources (i.e., Oral and Maxillofacial Surgery, Oncology, Otolaryngology).

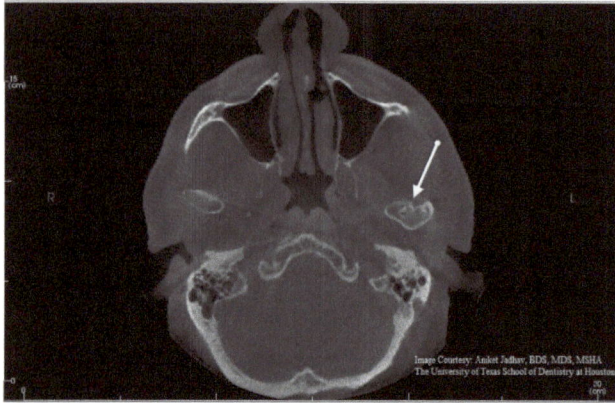

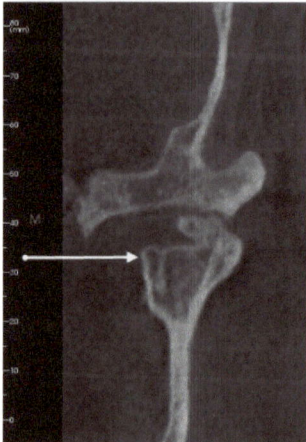

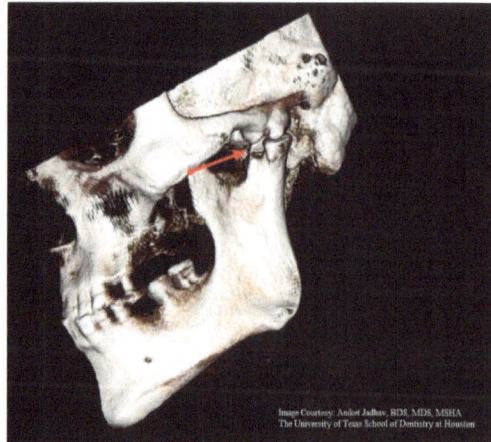

Figure 4-2, 3, and 4: *CBCT Images of a patient with Osteochondroma of left condyle (arrows): Courtesy of Aniket Jadhav, BDS, MDS, Department of Diagnostic and Biomedical Silences, The University of Texas School of Dentistry at Houston*

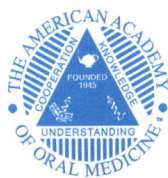

5 Sleep Disorders and Chronic Orofacial Pain

Common sleep disorders associated with chronic oral pain and general management guidelines are described below. Topics include sleep-related bruxism (SB) and the effect of orofacial pain on sleep quality. The term *sleep related* is used instead of *nocturnal* to include the activities and abnormalities that can occur with daytime sleep. There is presently no scientific documentation of a relationship connecting bruxism and articular disorders of the temporomandibular complex.

SLEEP-RELATED BRUXISM

- Defined as a parafunctional activity that includes clenching, bracing, gnashing, and grinding of the teeth
- Described in a more restricted way as orofacial motor activity during sleep, characterized by repetitive (phasic) or sustained (tonic) contractions of the jaw-closing muscles (i.e., the masseter and temporalis muscles)
- Associated with tooth-grinding sounds (otherwise, the condition is nonspecific)
- Prevalence of SB in the general population ranges from 6 to 8% and decreases rapidly with age (14% in childhood to 3% > 60 years of age)
- No gender predilection
- One of five sleep bruxers report concomitant orofacial pain
- Brain chemistry (e.g., dopaminergic sensitivity) has also been associated with bruxism
- SB may be linked to factors such as (1) lightening of sleep (i.e., micro-arousals), (2) rapid and transient electromyographic (EMG) leg/body activity, (3) short electrocardiographic increases in heart rate, and (4) frequent sleep stage shifts

Dental Management

From a clinical perspective, the recognition of SB by the dentist is based on the combined presence of two major subjective observations:

- A current history of tooth grinding or tapping sounds (not snoring) as confirmed by a bed partner
- The detection of abnormal tooth-wear facets that are not compatible with a history of normal (functional) wear

In addition, one or more of the following signs and symptoms may be reported concurrently:
- Temple headache
- Jaw muscle stiffness and limited range of motion or fatigue on awakening during the night or in the morning

Several methods are accessible to record and document the motor activity associated with SB. Electronics such as home audio and video recorders as well as portable (ambulatory) recording devices and comprehensive sleep laboratory (polysomnography) recorders may be used for confirmation to sleep parafunctional activities related to bruxism.

New research diagnostic criteria for the SB studies are proposed. According to these criteria, which are based on polysomnography and ambulatory recordings, SB is considered present on recognition of one of the following recording patterns:
- More than four episodes of rhythmic masticatory muscle activity (RMMA) per hour of sleep
- More than 25 bursts of RMMA per hour of sleep. Overnight, at least two grinding events should be observed.
- EMG threshold > 10% of maximal "awake" voluntary contraction with a duration of > 3 seconds and < 5 seconds between events
- Concomitant to SB, heart rate increase of at least 5% per minute

Since there is no specific cure for SB, the role of the health care clinician is to correctly manage these patients. The main goal should be the prevention of damage to the orofacial structures. The different types of intervention can be divided into three groups: behavioral, orthopedic, and pharmacologic treatments. So far, controlled studies that confirm the efficacy of behavior and pharmacologic strategies are lacking. However, a recent study demonstrated promise for clonidine with regard to therapeutic management of bruxism. Some of the recommendations in Table 5-1 directly address the patient's awareness of the disorder and his or her control of behaviors that are related to stress and anxiety.

OROFACIAL PAIN AND SLEEP PROBLEMS

It is not uncommon for patients with orofacial muscle pain to report poor sleep quality. However, rarely do TMD patients wake up in pain during their sleep. Unlike dental pain associated with pulpitis, which can delay sleep onset or interrupt ongoing sleep, conditions such as osteoarthritis of the temporomandibular joint or trigeminal neuralgia seldom interfere with sleep.

DENTAL MANAGEMENT

The most common complaints of patients suffering from myofascial pain indicative of poor sleep are restlessness, unrefreshing sleep, not enough sleep, light sleep, disrupted sleep, and unrestorative sleep. Concomitantly, these patients may report excessive daytime fatigue, irritable bowels, and poor resistance to stress. The use of a diary to rate pain in relation to sleep habits (e.g., bedtime, sleep latency, sleep duration) and diurnal activities (e.g., time and type of meal, stress factors) is sometimes helpful to characterize the ongoing patterns and contributing factors.

The polysomnography observations of reduced sleep duration, an increase in the number of awakenings and body movements, and reduced duration of sleep stages 3 and 4 are common in the "poor" sleeper, both with and without pain. The presence of alpha-electric cortical activity on the electroencephalogram, described as an intrusion of "awake" brain activity, has been associated with fibromyalgia and arthritis. However, the specificity of this phenomenon in relation to pain remains to be assessed because it has also been observed in several other medical (e.g., depression, sleep apnea, periodic myoclonus) and environmental (e.g., noise or excessive heat in the bedroom) conditions. However, masticatory muscle pain in bruxers is not associated with sleep disruption or a complaint of poor sleep quality.

TABLE 5–1: BEHAVIORAL STRATEGIES/TREATMENT MODALITIES*
Wind down during the second half of the evening. Rest 60–90 minutes before bedtime; avoid intense thinking, discussions, or action; separate body and mind from day's activities.
Learn a relaxation technique (e.g., "conscious" respiration) and practice it during the day and before bedtime (psychologists and physical therapists can help patients master this strategy)
Maintain a good physical condition to feel healthier (avoid extensive exercise after 6 pm)
Avoid copious meals and beverages such as coffee, tea, soft drinks, and alcohol (limited intake around dinner time: stop intake in the evening, approximately 3 hours before bedtime)
Stop smoking after 7 pm because nicotine is known to increase muscle tone and arousal
Create a good sleeping hygiene environment with a comfortable bed and mattress in a quiet room (hamper external sounds; use ear plugs when the bed partner snores or makes any disrupting sounds while asleep; adjust the temperature to about 65°F [18°C]; allow incoming fresh air)
Couples with an infant should make arrangements to get at least a few nights of undisturbed sleep per week. Further management strategies include biofeedback and hypnosis. Biofeedback appliances that use an audio signal or a small electrical stimulus have been applied for the short-term management of sleep- related bruxism (SB).
Hypnosis, which is considered a form of relaxation therapy, has been reported to aid certain patients
Occlusal appliances (see Chapter 4, "Temporomandibular Disorders: Myogenous and Arthrogenous Conditions") such as a mouth guard may protect further injury to tooth and periodontal structures
Pharmacologic treatment is indicated for use cautiously on a short-term basis only. Drugs such as benzodiazepines, muscle relaxants, and tricyclic antidepressants (TCAs) have been suggested. However, TCAs did not show efficacy for SB.

*Adapted from Zarcone VP

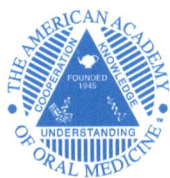

6 Cancer and Chronic Orofacial Pain

Orofacial and head and neck pain can arise because of malignant disease or the management of cancer. This pain is affected by significant psychosocial issues that surround malignant disease. Whenever possible, recognition of all factors leading to the pain or stomatitis should be addressed. Symptom management is needed until pain is controlled.

Pain from a tumor may be due to pressure, necrosis, inflammation, mucosal ulceration, nerve compression or invasion, and altered function caused by tissue invasion that can lead to muscle spasm. Pain management often requiring systemic analgesics (see below) is required while treatment of the malignant disease is initiated.

MUCOSITIS
The incidence and severity of mucositis have been related to the nature of cancer treatment, including but not limited to radiation therapy to head and neck and the degree of preexisting mucosal disease, and to oral hygiene.

Therapies include the following:
- Bland rinses (0.9% saline solutions with or without sodium bicarbonate), topical anesthetics, mucosal coating agents (Milk of Magnesia, kaolin-pectin, Amphogel, and sucralfate)
- Topical anesthetics/analgesics: Benadryl, dyclonine, and viscous lidocaine (may cause burning, especially on ulcerated mucosa; may eliminate taste and cause the loss of the gag reflex and increase the risk of aspiration), topical morphine, and doxepin suspension
- Systemic agents (see below) may be needed in addition to topical anesthetic/ analgesic agents

ORAL INFECTIONS
Patients should be evaluated for dental and periodontal disease before the initiation of cancer therapy. Reactivation of viral infection is common in myelosuppressed or immunosuppressed patients (Table 6-1). Candidiasis and other fungal infections and periodontal and pulpal infections may present in oncology patients. Further, mucositis and secondary infection after chemotherapy and/or radiation therapy also present in these patients. (See *Clinician's Guide to Diagnosis and Treatment of Common Oral Conditions*.) Maintaining good oral hygiene may reduce oral mucositis and decrease the risk of local infection.

TABLE 6 – 1: ORAL VIRAL INFECTIONS AND THERAPIES	
Virus	*Therapy*
Herpes simplex virus infection	Acyclovir therapy/valacyclovir therapy
Varicella zoster virus infection	Acyclovir/valacyclovir/famotidine therapy

MUSCULOSKELETAL PAIN
Musculoskeletal syndromes are commonly seen in patients with head and neck cancer. The etiology of dysfunction includes the direct effects of the tumor on muscles, on bone destruction, and on pathologic fractures. The effects of surgical treatment may be significant if discontinuity of the jaw or fibrosis of muscles and the soft tissue occurs. Radiation fibrosis of the muscles and soft tissue and complications of osteoradionecrosis may affect jaw function. The altered function of the mandible may place stress on the temporomandibular joint or the muscles of mastication, resulting in further dysfunction and pain. The pain experience is conditioned by stress, anxiety, and depression associated with cancer that may increase the difficulty of management. Reduction of salivary gland secretions complicates physical condition further more.

MANAGEMENT
- Referral to physical therapy
- Force fluid might be necessary
- Fabrication of guidance appliance or orthotic/ occlusal appliance

- Anti-inflammatory agents/analgesics, muscle relaxants
- Tricyclic antidepressants/antiseizure medications (see sections on postherpetic neuralgia and burning mouth syndrome)
- Referral to Oral Medicine, oncologist, or physician for pain management

NECROSIS

The initial treatment of post-radiation osteonecrosis, or necrosis associated with bisphosphonates includes maintenance of good oral hygiene, antiseptic rinses, and antibiotics to reduce/control secondary bacterial irritation, and appropriate pain management. Control of pain often requires the use of systemic analgesics. Resolution of the lesion may require referral to Oral and Maxillofacial Surgery for hyperbaric oxygen therapy and/or surgery, for post-radiation osteonecrosis, but it has not been shown effective in bisphosphonate necrosis.

NEUROLOGIC PAIN

Neurologic pain in the head and neck cancer patient may arise from traumatic neuroma, somatic and autonomic collateralization, and/or deafferenation following surgery. Chemotherapy-induced pain and neuralgia-like pain or neuropathy can develop following chemotherapy and surgical treatment; neuropathic pain resulting in aching or burning discomfort may develop between episodes of the electric-like pain or be experienced on a chronic basis (see Chapter 1, "Oral Neuropathic Pain Conditions," for further information).

SYSTEMIC MEDICATIONS IN PAIN MANAGEMENT

Medications used in the treatment of cancer pain may be divided into those directed at the cancer or at the complications of its treatment that are causing pain and palliative therapy directed at symptom control. Those that modify the cause of pain include anti-infective, anti-inflammatory, and anticonvulsant drugs and analgesics. Analgesics are more effective, and a lower total dose is needed when the medication is provided on a time-contingent basis. Drug interactions and the status of liver and kidney function must be considered in the choice and dose regimens of medications. A major problem in the use of analgesics in cancer patients is the reluctance of health care providers to provide adequate dosages and frequency to effectively control pain. The use of opioids in cancer (and other) patients with severe pain does not tend to result in difficulties with narcotic addiction.

BEHAVIORAL APPROACHES AND SUPPORTIVE CARE

Management of pain may require the use of psychological and physical therapies. Relaxation, imagery, biofeedback, hypnosis, transcutaneous electric nerve stimulation, and other therapies have been applied in the management of cancer pain. (See Appendix IV, "Referral in the Management of Chronic Orofacial Pain Disorders.")

SUMMARY AND CONCLUSIONS

Orofacial pain occurs in patients with head and neck cancer. It is a complication of the medical management in patients who receive aggressive chemotherapy protocols and in the majority of those who receive bone marrow and stem cell transplantation and neutropenia-inducing cancer therapy. The significance of pain in the head and neck region can be magnified because of the importance of the region in growth and development and psychological and social interactions. Management strategies for oral and maxillofacial cancer pain are based on principles of management of acute and chronic pain. Awareness of the medical and dental conditions and knowledge of the effects of the cancer treatment are necessary to understand the multiple causes of pain and to select therapy.

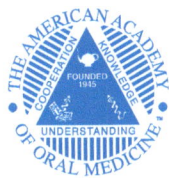

Appendix I

Taking A History for the Chronic Orofacial Pain Patient*

The diagnosis of chronic orofacial pain may present a challenge to the clinician because there may be no clinical signs of disease present to aid in the diagnostic process or a known cause cannot be effectively managed (e.g., cancer, chronic pain due to herpetic neuralgia). Crucial and often underappreciated is the need to obtain a complete history. This should include the patient's chief complaint, a history of the present illness (history of the chief complaint), a review of systems, family and social history, and a psychological screening. Many medical history forms are commercially available that provide a guide for a review of systems. Special emphasis should be placed on disorders involving the head, face, eyes, ears, nose, neck, and throat since disorders affecting any of these areas may be the source of the patient's complaint. The astute clinician must also consider systemic disorders that can cause or exacerbate facial pain or dysfunction.

CHIEF COMPLAINT

The chief complaint should be recorded in the patient's own words so that the clinician can attempt to communicate with the patient at a mutual level of understanding. The chief complaint is not the diagnosis rather it is a subjective finding. Often the patient may believe that he or she has a particular diagnostic entity, which may reflect another health practitioner's opinion and may or may not have validity. It is important for each clinician to determine an independent diagnosis. Significance of chronologic history of past treatment provided either succeeded or failed should be taken into considerations.

It is important to evaluate the patient's report of the chief complaint. This is accomplished by careful and specific questioning to direct the interview such that all of the necessary information regarding the patient's symptoms of pain will be obtained. A number of fill-in-the-blanks forms have been developed for chronic orofacial pain patients; however, there is no substitute for using open-ended questioning.

HISTORY OF PRESENT ILLNESS

Chronology: date of onset; time of day the pain occurs; progression of pain after onset; duration, frequency, and referral pattern of the symptoms; previous episodes of similar pain; constant or intermittent; temporal associations

Character (pain descriptors, qualitative aspect): dull, aching, tightness, pressure, throbbing, pulsing, pounding, sharp, shooting, lancinating, electric shock-like, and burning

Location (static or migratory): pain should correspond to the anatomic distribution of the nerves in the involved area

Intensity (quantitative): mild, moderate, severe, excruciating, intractable. May use a 0-10 Numeric Rating Scale

Frequency: how often does the pain occur

Duration: how long does the pain last

Chronicity: pain lasting more than 3 months

Associated signs or symptoms: visual aura, autonomic, nervous system manifestations, systemic signs or symptoms

Aggravating factors: what makes the pain worse?

Alleviating factors: what makes the pain better

Previous treatment: note both successful and unsuccessful treatments. In the case of medications, take note of the relief provided, if any, dose, dosing interval, side effects and how long the medication trial was.

Other: family history; trauma history; precipitating factors; aggravating factors; what provides relief of pain; previous diagnostic tests and results; previous treatment and effectiveness; diet

---

* Adapted with permission from Balciunas BA, Siegel MA, Grace EG. A clinical approach to the diagnosis of facial pain. *Dent Clin North Am* 1992; 36:987–1000.

SYSTEMIC DISORDERS AND ASSOCIATED FACIAL PAIN/DYSFUNCTION

Cardiovascular System
- Hypertension
- Vascular headaches
- Ischemic heart disease
- Referred pain to the left mandible/molars

Central Nervous System
- Multiple sclerosis
- Facial paralysis/paresthesia
- Trigeminal neuralgia
- Myasthenia gravis
- Facial muscle weakness
- Psychological or psychiatric disorders
- Chronic facial pain, chronic headaches

Connective Tissue Disorders
- Arthritis
- Occipital headaches, temporomandibular joint (TMJ) involvement/temporomandibular disorder (TMD)
- Fibromyalgia
- Myalgia, TMD involvement
- Systemic lupus erythematosus
- Temporal arteritis
- Headaches, jaw claudication pain
- Scleroderma
- Paresthesia

Endocrine
- Hypoglycemia
- Vascular headaches
- Hyperglycemia
- Diabetic neuropathy, burning mouth syndrome, xerostomia
- Hypothyroidism
- Chronic muscle fatigue, vascular headaches
- Subacute thyroiditis
- Ear pain, referred pain to left mandible, sore throat

Musculoskeletal
- Cervical spine disorders
- Headaches
- Upper quadrant dysfunction
- Facial pain
- Calcified stylohyoid ligament

SIGNS AND SYMPTOMS NECESSITATING EMERGENCY REFERRAL

1. Headache of acute onset associated with neurologic symptoms
2. Headache described as "worst headache of my life"
3. Headache of acute onset accompanied by neck stiffness, fever, and vomiting
4. Loss of consciousness or seizures accompanying headache
5. Significant change in headache pattern
6. SNOOP, systemic symptoms, neurological signs and symptoms, onset, older age, past headache history

TABLE I–1: ONSET CHARACTERISTICS	
Age	*Differential Diagnosis*
Childhood through age 30 yrs	Migraine headaches
Late 20s to early 30s	Cluster headaches
Between the ages of 20 and 40 yrs	Temporomandibular disorder and tension headaches
Over age 50 yrs	Glossopharyngeal neuralgia, postherpetic neuralgia, temporal arteritis, trigeminal neuralgia
Any age	Pain that is related to a traumatic or stressful episode

TABLE I–2: TIME OF DAY	
Time	*Differential Diagnosis*
12 am to 4 am	Cluster headaches
Occurs on awakening	Hypertension headaches, migraine headaches, nocturnal bruxism
During the morning	Frontal sinus pain
During the afternoon	Maxillary sinus pain
End of the day	Tension headaches

TABLE 1-3: CHRONICITY	
Duration	**Differential Diagnosis**
Acute	Acute sinusitis, intracranial disorder, temporal arteritis
Chronic intermittent	Migraine headaches, cluster headaches, glossopharyngeal neuralgia, sinus pain, trigeminal neuralgia
Chronic persistent	Atypical facial pain, temporomandibular disorder, tension headaches
Cyclic	Related to hormone cycles, diurnal rhythm, etc.

TABLE 1-4: DEGREE OF PAIN	
Pain Descriptor	**Differential Diagnosis**
Excruciating	Cerebrovascular disease, cluster headaches
Severe	Acute sinusitis, glossopharyngeal neuralgia, hypertension headaches, migraine headaches, post-herpetic neuralgia, temporal arteritis, trigeminal neuralgia
Moderate	Atypical facial pain, chronic sinusitis, muscular temporomandibular disorder, tension headaches

TABLE 1-5: QUALITY	
Pain Descriptor	**Differential Diagnosis**
Throbbing, pounding, or pulsing	Cluster headaches, hypertension headaches, migraine headaches, severe acute sinusitis, vascular pain
Dull, aching, tightness, or pressure	Bruxism, temporomandibular disorder, chronic sinus pain, clenching, toothache
Sharp, shooting, lancinating, or electric shock	Glossopharyngeal neuralgia, trigeminal neuralgia
Burning or aching	Atypical facial pain, reflex sympathetic dystrophy, muscle tension headache, postherpetic neuralgia
Numbness, tingling, or paresthesia	Facial myospasm, tension headaches, cervical nerve compression, scleroderma, malignancy

PROGRESSION

- Does anything make the pain better?
- Does anything make the pain worse?
- Does the pain get better throughout the day?
- Does the pain get worse throughout the day?
- What effect have previous treatments had?
- Does the weather affect the condition?
- Do either hot or cold affect the condition?

FAMILY HISTORY

A family history may elucidate either systemic disease states that may be inherited or traits that may have a tendency to run in families. Questions that ascertain the health of parents, grandparents, siblings, and offspring may prove helpful. If the patient's relatives are deceased, the cause of death may offer further information.

SOCIAL AND PSYCHOLOGICAL HISTORY

Following the initial formulation of a differential diagnosis, a social and psychological history should be reviewed. Typical social history questions will probe the patient's lifestyle regarding avocation, habits, relationships, drug use and abuse, including alcohol and tobacco use, hobbies, and travel. Some standard questions can be used as a guide for determining whether additional psychological testing is necessary. (See Appendix II.)

After initial questioning, patients may correct, embellish, or add to their previous answers. Patients may initially deny conditions such as stress, depression, physical or drug abuse, and anxiety when these conditions are evident from other aspects of the history. After repeating the same question in a variety of ways, the answer may change.

Thus, the importance of interviewing versus handing out and collecting forms is underscored.

After completing a thorough evaluation of the medical history and a detailed review of the patient's chief complaint, the practitioner will generally be able to formulate a differential diagnosis. The clinical and physical examinations, along with diagnostic testing, can further direct the clinician toward formulating a working diagnosis from which therapy can be initiated.

TABLE I–6: LOCATION	
Location	**Differential Diagnosis**
Cervical	Arthritis, carotodynia, tension headache
Frontal	Cluster headaches, migraine headaches, sinus headaches, muscle tension headaches, ocular disorders, post-herpetic neuralgia
Mandible	Atypical facial pain, glossopharyngeal neuralgia, referred pain of cardiac origin, subacute thyroiditis, trigeminal neuralgia, reflex sympathetic dystrophy
Maxilla	Atypical facial pain, lesions in the maxillary sinus, sinusitis, trigeminal neuralgia
Nasal/paranasal	Glossopharyngeal neuralgia, sinusitis, trigeminal neuralgia, postherpetic neuralgia
Occipital	Cervical arthritis, hypertensive headache, muscle tension headache
Orbital	Cluster headache, migraine headache, ocular and/or optic disorders, postherpetic neuralgia, sinusitis
Temporal	Hypertension headache, migraine headache, postherpetic neuralgia, temporal arteritis, temporomandibular disorder
Throat	Carotodynia, glossopharyngeal neuralgia, subacute thyroiditis

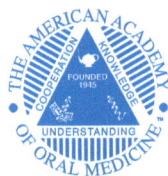

Appendix II
Psychological Aspects of Chronic Orofacial Pain

The interrelationship between chronic orofacial pain and psychological, psychosocial, and behavioral factors is complex. Depression may be either primary or secondary; it may be an initiating factor in the patient's chronic pain condition, or the chronic pain condition may be a factor relating to the patient's depression. Chronic orofacial pain, like other chronic pain states, such as headache and back pain may be associated with significant disability days, depression, and frequent pain visits. In addition, stress may play a role in either the initiation or promotion of chronic orofacial pain through a variety of mechanisms that include activation of the hypothalamic-pituitary-adrenal axis, up regulation of the sympathetic nervous system, and secondary effects on sleep and parafunctional behavior. Consequently, it is important for the clinician evaluating patients with chronic orofacial pain to assess for psychological, psychosocial, and behavioral factors that may be contributory and responsive to appropriate referral.

A number of self-report measurement instruments have been published that may be useful in assessing the patient's psychosocial status. These include the Minnesota Multiphasic Personality Inventory (MMPI), the Symptom Checklist-90 revised (SCL-90R), The TMJ Scale, the IMPATH Scale for TMDs, the Multidimensional Pain Inventory (MPI), and the Graded Chronic Pain Scale, among others. Many of these scales not only quantify pain but help in defining the level to which pain is disabling. Several axis II (psychological and emotional axis) assessment forms available through www.rdc-tmdinternational.org to down load and use (see Ohrbach et al. in reference list).

On the other hand, several screening questions may provide an insight into the patient's psychological state. A significant number of positive responses to the following questions may mandate referral for a psychological evaluation:
- Are you experiencing stress at the present time? If so, what do you believe is causing the stress?
- Have you experienced any major life change in the past 2 years? If so, is there a time relationship with this change and your painful condition?
- Have you had any significant work-related changes?
- Are you more tired than you should be with respect to the amount of time you are working and the amount of sleep you are getting?
- Are you having any problems falling asleep or staying asleep?
- Are you depressed or anxious? Have you had any feelings of self-doubt or thoughts of suicide?
- Have there been any recent deaths or serious illnesses in your family?
- Do you consider yourself a perfectionist in any aspect of your life?
- Does the pain or discomfort interfere with your ability to work and/or perform your usual daily tasks?
- Have you or has anyone in your family experienced physical, drug, or emotional abuse?
- Have you at present or in the past (or anyone in your family) participated in psychological or psychiatric counseling?
- Why do you think you have this pain problem?
- What do you do to cope with your pain?
- How much time do you spend sitting or lying down because of the pain condition?

Patients with presumed psychological conditions beyond the expertise of the clinician should be referred to appropriate resources. A recent study reported a positive correlation between low self-esteem, feeling worried, low energy and sleep activity (each is a correlate of depression), and treatment failure in patients with temporomandibular disorder. Therefore, referral to appropriate resources for depressed patients with chronic orofacial pain may be beneficial. (See Appendix IV) This is particularly meaningful since the prognosis is often worse when the patient's biomedical status is confounded by comorbid psychological and psychosocial abnormalities. Also, referral should be considered for patients who do not respond to appropriate treatment or who request invasive intervention without objective evidence of disease. Often physicians and dentists err by over escalating therapy in an attempt to eliminate pain with ablative surgical procedures or inappropriate drug therapy. For these patients, referral to multidisciplinary pain centers is indicated.

The clinician treating the chronic orofacial pain patient must be aware of the psychological and psychosocial aspects of patient management. Biobehavioral treatment of chronic pain is typically based on a rehabilitation model that incorporates self-management skills and other approaches that include education, behavioral modification (e.g., cessation of daytime clenching, fingernail biting, anterior jaw posturing), biofeedback, imagery, relaxation therapy, coping mechanisms, hypnosis, and other cognitive-behavioral therapies. It is critical for the clinician to appreciate the importance of the psychological, psychosocial, and biobehavioral influences on chronic orofacial pain and treatment perspectives. Further, there is immense value in a positive caring attitude as the placebo effect has the potential to benefit almost any therapy.

Appendix III

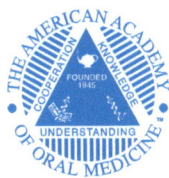

Diagnostic Imaging and Chronic Orofacial Pain

One of the requirements for successful management of patients with chronic orofacial pain is the collection of sufficient diagnostic information to lead to the proper diagnosis and treatment. The information needed may or may not include imaging. In deciding when, or even whether, to obtain diagnostic imaging, clinicians must first determine what type of information is needed to diagnose the condition and manage the patient appropriately and whether imaging is the best source of that data. They then must decide which imaging technique will provide that knowledge in the most cost-effective manner, without unnecessary patient expense or radiation exposure.

The goals of imaging in general are to evaluate the integrity of structures when disease is suspected, to confirm the extent of known disease, to rule out or rule in particular diagnostic entities, to stage the progression of known disease, and to evaluate the effects of treatment. For the patient with chronic orofacial pain, the systems imaged may include the teeth and supporting bone, the hard and soft tissues of the temporomandibular joint (TMJ), the paranasal sinuses, and other structures of the head and neck, depending on the nature and location of symptoms.

Although there are published guidelines for selecting radiologic examinations for patients with a variety of needs, including the new and recall dental patient, selection criteria for chronic orofacial pain have not yet been established. Selection criteria are those clinical signs

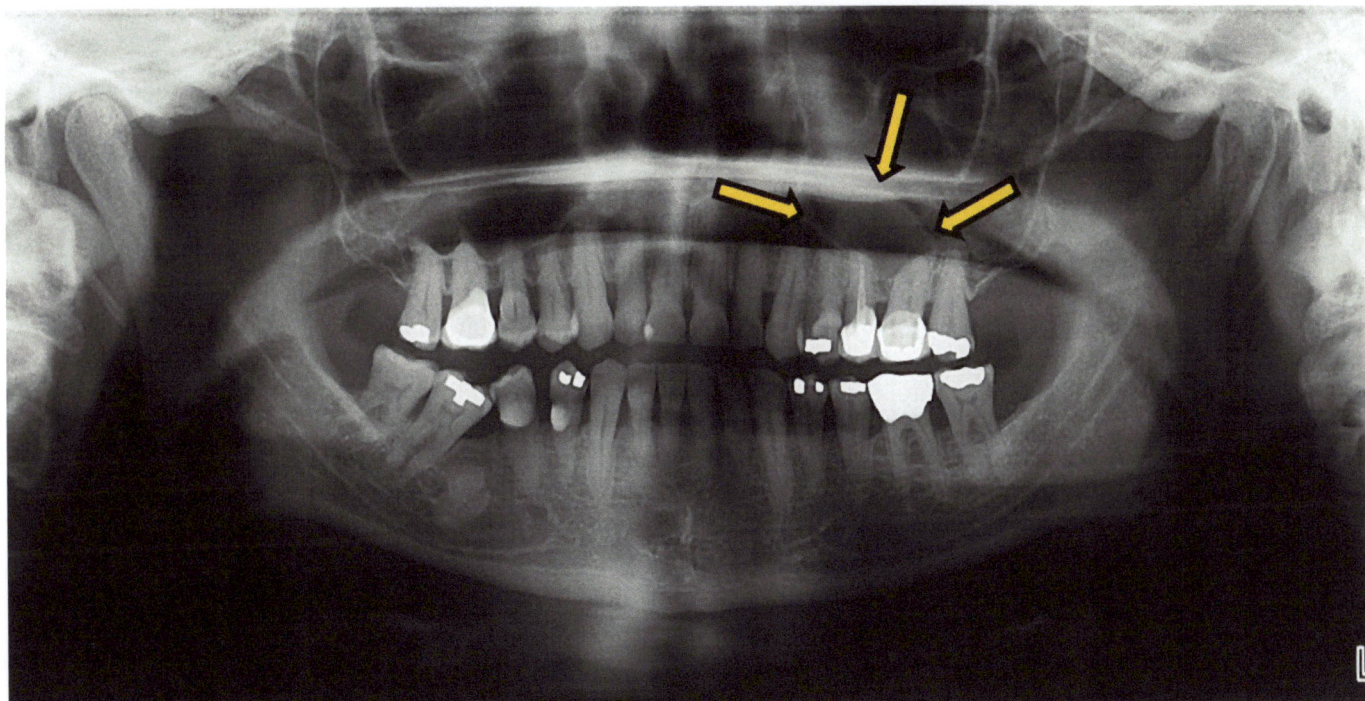

Figure III-1 *Image of Chronic Sinusitis with Pseudocyst of left sinus (arrows)* — courtesy of Shawn Adibi, DDS, MEd, Department of General Practice and Dental Public Health, The University of Texas School of Dentistry at Houston

TABLE III-1: EVALUATION OF IMAGING TECHNIQUES	
Advantages	**Disadvantages**
Panoramic: low cost; provides adequate view of both jaws, good overall view	Oblique view; only gross structural changes observable; only shows lateral and central portions of condyles (see example)
Transcranial: moderate cost; good view of the lateral portion of the temporomandibular joint	Medial and central portions of the condyle are positioned downward; the outline of the condyle and fossa tends to be distorted (structural relationships are difficult to interpret)
Conventional tomography: moderate cost; good detail or osseous structures in entire joint	No information on soft tissue; cannot reliably determine disk position from condylar position
Computed tomography (CT): provides fine detail about osseous structures; can demonstrate all portions of the jointwell	Expensive, higher radiation dose required (should be reserved for situations in which fine detail is required, such as suspected tumors, ankylosis, complex facial fractures, or foreign body giant cell reactions to implants)
Cone-beam computed tomography: provides fine detail of osseous structures; images reconstructed into multiplanar and three-dimensional rendering to view joint from all aspects; lower radiation dose and generally lower cost than CT	New technology that is not available everywhere; no soft tissue information
Arthrography: can evaluate the joint in motion; provides access for lavage	Expensive, invasive
Magnetic resonance imaging: good visualization of all portions of soft tissue areas; shows location and condition of disk	Expensive; requires patient confinement during procedure; not indicated for patients with pacemakers

and symptoms that suggest that a radiologic examination would contribute to the proper diagnosis and management of the condition. The most appropriate imaging procedures are those that provide new information that will influence patient care. The imaging examination should be selected only after a review of the clinical and historical findings, the clinical diagnosis, the results of prior imaging studies, the tentative treatment plan, the cost of the examination, and the radiation dose.

For chronic orofacial pain that does not appear to be related to the TMJ or associated structures, the clinician usually needs to rule out a dental cause of the pain before exploring other non-dental causes. Intraoral and/or panoramic radiographs, depending on the specific problem being explored may be appropriate in this situation. When maxillary sinusitis is suspected as the cause of the pain, the patient should be referred either to an otolaryngologist or to a hospital radiology department for a complete sinus assessment, which is usually accomplished with a computed tomographic (CT) examination. Suspicion of a central lesion, such as a neoplasm, calls for

further evaluation, including CT and perhaps magnetic resonance imaging (MRI). Selection of imaging technique may require a consultation.

When the chronic facial pain appears to be associated with the TMJ, the clinician must decide whether knowledge of hard and/or soft tissue abnormalities will be useful in the management of the patient. There is little correlation between the clinical and radiologic findings in temporomandibular disorders. There is also conflicting information in the literature about the usefulness of tomography in the management of these patients. However, if the clinician feels that information about the osseous tissues is needed, a wide choice of imaging modalities is available. The condition of the condyle, glenoid fossa, and articular eminence can be determined with varying degrees of detail from panoramic radiographs, a wide variety of plain films, transcranial projections, conventional tomography, CT, and cone-beam CT. The major differences between these imaging systems are in the amount of bony detail they can provide, the thoroughness with which they cover the joint, and the cost of the examination. Further, MRI may be useful in the evaluation of connective tissues such as the disk.

CONCLUSION

The choice of imaging procedure, if any, belongs to the clinician who is ultimately responsible for the care of the patient. However, the type of information needed, the detail required, and the potential impact of this information on patient management should be the prime determinants in selecting the diagnostic examination. If a positive or negative result does not affect management, there is little rationale for ordering such an imaging study. A more in-depth discussion of TMJ imaging can be found in the position paper of the American Academy of Oral and Maxillofacial Radiology.

Appendix IV

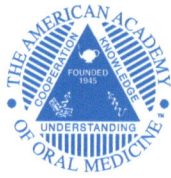

Referral In the Management of Chronic Orofacial Pain Disorders

When to refer is an issue that is faced by all practitioners involved in the diagnosis and treatment of orofacial pain (OFP) disorders. OFP is a symptom that may be difficult to diagnose and manage, with multiple potential causes such as regional disease of the head and neck, a generalized musculoskeletal or rheumatic disorder, peripheral or central nervous system disease, or a psychological abnormality. These patients are challenging for the diagnosis and treatment and often require additional training and expertise for management that may be beyond the scope of general practitioners. The challenge is obvious when considering the large number of conditions that present as OFP. Ethics requires that dentists provide treatment only when qualified by training or experience; otherwise, a consultation and/or referral to an appropriate practitioner is warranted.

REASONS FOR REFERRAL
- The dentist's skill and/or interest in the specific disorder is limited.
- The dentist's relationship with the patient is a problem.
- Specialized expertise is required.
- Referral to a dental or medical specialist when a diagnosis is unknown or suspected but not established. This referral may be to order diagnostic or confirming tests such as laboratory or imaging studies.
- Referral to a dental specialist after a diagnosis is made and the practitioner is not comfortable providing the treatment or chooses not to provide treatment.
- Referral to a dental or medical specialist when the diagnosis is known but the condition is not ordinarily treated by the practitioner (e.g., trigeminal neuralgia).
- Referral to another clinician when a second opinion is requested.

The dentist's first responsibility is diagnostic: to rule out/ in odontogenic pain/conditions and to identify complaints arising from orofacial structures that are correctable through dental therapy. When this cannot be done, it is the dentist's responsibility to refer the patient to a competent clinician or specialist.

Decisions about referral rely on the ability to recognize the OFP disorders that one can competently treat alone, those that require consultation and collaboration with others, and those that are better managed by others.

DENTAL DISCIPLINES AND MEDICAL SPECIALTIES COMMONLY INVOLVED IN DIAGNOSIS AND MANAGEMENT OF OROFACIAL PAIN:

Dental Disciplines
Endodontists primarily diagnose and treat pulpal disease, which usually presents with pain as a dominant symptom. Root fractures, internal and external resorption, partially necrotic pulp disease, failed endodontics, possible pulpal disease in connection with maxillary sinusitis, pulpal disease in combination with periodontal disease, and pulpal disease under fixed prosthetics may require special expertise to diagnose and treat. Referral to an endodontist may be made to evaluate a patient to differentiate between pain of pulpal origin and atypical facial pain.

Oral Medicine provides the diagnosis and physical and medical management of such painful conditions as chronic inflammatory disorders of the oral mucosa, difficult oral or dental diagnoses, oral manifestations of systemic disease, dental management of the medically complex patient, and oral behavioral, musculoskeletal, and neurologic/neuropathic pain disorders and pain associated with systemic disease and medical management. Diagnosis may involve ordering of medical laboratory and advanced medical imaging, soft tissue biopsy, and other diagnostic tests.

Oral and maxillofacial radiologists are involved in the diagnosis of many painful oral conditions with reference to imaging. Magnetic resonance imaging, computed tomography, cone-beam computed tomography, arthrography, radioisotope imaging, and conventional tomography are some of the intraoral and extraoral radiologic techniques that may be employed to aid in the diagnosis of painful orofacial conditions. These services may also be provided by a medical radiologist.

Oral and maxillofacial surgeons diagnose and treat infections, trauma, cysts, and tumors of the jaws. In some instances surgical management is considered but must be based upon specific patient findings or specific findings on diagnostic testing. Surgery is rarely considered in musculo-skeletal conditions, including temporomandibular disorder (TMD), and in neurologic and neuropathic pain states. Surgical options such as arthrocentesis (lavage), arthroscopy, or open temporomandibular joint (TMJ) surgery should be considered only in TMD cases that meet very specific criteria (i.e., chronic intractable joint pain, demonstrable TMJ pathology, poor response to conservative therapy, and psychological stability). Arthrocentesis has been advocated for specific TMDs such as sudden-onset severe closed lock and severe limited mouth opening. Arthroscopy provides a window to visualize intra-articular structures and operate with minimal trauma within the capsule. Both arthrocentesis and arthroplasty are now rarely considered and require postoperative physical therapy and rehabilitation. On even more rare occasions, open TMJ surgery may be necessary in the repair of degenerative processes of the glenoid fossa, condylar head, and/or meniscus. The role of surgery has decreased in the management of TMDs but nonetheless continues to play a limited but important role.

Orofacial Pain specialists serve as a consultant to other dentists, physicians and other healthcare providers, but is frequently the principal treating health care provider administering care at various levels. The scope of care includes the diagnosis and treatment of systemic disorders that cause orofacial pain, masticatory and cervical musculoskeletal pain, neurovascular pain, neuropathic pain, sleep disorders related to orofacial pain and orofacial movement disorders.

Other disciplines of dentistry, including orthodontics, periodontics, prosthodontics, pediatric dentistry, and general dentistry, may have advanced training and experience with respect to the diagnosis and management of chronic orofacial pain.

MEDICAL SPECIALTIES

Allergists and dermatologists. The diagnosis and management of contact or other hypersensitivity reactions may require a consultation with an allergist or dermatologist. The patient may be referred for standardized patch testing.

Anesthesiologists. These are the specialists who most commonly perform such procedures as sympathetic ganglion blocks (e.g., stellate ganglion block in the diagnosis and therapy of complex regional pain syndrome/reflex sympathetic dystrophy), other local anesthesia procedures, and pharmacotherapeutics strategies for chronic pain. Multidisciplinary chronic pain centers may be managed by anesthesiologists.

Gastroenterology. Gastric reflux and dental erosion leading to dental sensitivity require referral for diagnosis and treatment. Disorders associated with regurgitation may be associated with eating disorders or diseases of the stomach and esophagus. In patients with dental erosion secondary to gastric reflux, it is necessary to control the medical condition before restoring the dentition.

Internal medicine/primary care. It is important for patients to have a primary care physician as a general resource. The primary care physician can provide a thorough medical assessment to eliminate the possibility of undiscovered disease that may be contributing to pain. The physician can provide insight and support for psychosocial issues that may impact on the management of chronic OFP. The primary care physician becomes an important resource in difficult diagnostic and treatment situations. Often this primary care provider is an internist, but family or general medical practitioners, pediatricians, and gynecologists may act as primary care physicians.

Neurology. An ever-present concern is the possibility that OFP may be due to disease of the peripheral or central nervous system or invasion and destruction of nerves by tumor. For example, an acoustic neuroma occurring in the cerebellopontine region may cause facial pain associated with hearing loss. Trigeminal neuralgia, cluster headache, migraine, and its variants are commonly diagnosed and treated by neurologists. Movement disorders including tardive dyskinesia (often a side effect of long-term psychotropic and antiparkinsonian drugs) are associated with repetitive mouth movements that may lead to facial pain. In the treatment of these and other conditions, including neuralgias and chronic pain syndromes, it may be necessary to consult with or refer the patient to a neurologist.

Otolaryngology. The proximity of auditory organs and structures of the upper airway to the mouth creates a natural interdisciplinary alignment between dentistry and otolaryngology. Pulpal and periapical disease may manifest as sinus pain, and sinusitis will manifest as dental pain. Further, sinus disease and tumors of the nasopharynx and infratemporal fossa may present as chronic facial pain and necessitate referral between a dentist and an otolaryngologist.

Physical medicine (physiatrist) and rehabilitation. Masticatory muscle disorders and traumatic injury to temporomandibular structures may necessitate referral to or collaboration with a physiatrist. Patients may present with complaints of jaw pain and dysfunction that are part of a more generalized chronic musculoskeletal disorder. These patients may not respond well to local therapy for the jaw unless systemic management is provided. Physical medicine approaches to managing TMDs are considered important nonsurgical therapies. A physiatrist can offer advice regarding modalities of treatment or provide aspects of TMD treatment

Psychiatry/psychology. Chronic pain includes an emotional component with significant effects that must be addressed. The symptom of OFP may also be a manifestation of a psychiatric disorder. Dentists are not trained to diagnose or treat psychological disorders. However, dentists may play a role with proper referral for psychiatric and psychological evaluations. The patient's primary care physician is a valuable resource to discuss a possible referral for psychological assessment.

Rheumatology. Generalized arthritis and connective tissue disease (e.g., scleroderma, lupus, rheumatoid arthritis) may manifest with symptoms similar to TMD or nonspecific chronic pain of the oral and perioral regions. Conditions such as fibromyalgia, a chronic generalized musculoskeletal pain disorder, may present with symptoms of pain in the masticatory muscles and TMJ area. These conditions may necessitate referral between a dentist and a rheumatologist.

Multispecialty pain clinics. An interdisciplinary team approach in chronic pain management is invaluable. Combining diverse medical and dental disciplines, including but not limited to anesthesiology, neurology, psychiatry, psychology, physical medicine, rheumatology, surgery, radiology, general dentists, and dental specialists, has many advantages. Other health care professionals that are often part of interdisciplinary teams include physiotherapists, occupational therapists, and social workers.

SIGNS AND SYMPTOMS INDICATING A NEED FOR REFERRAL

As a general rule, any patient with OFP who has symptoms that cannot be explained by a dental etiology is a candidate for referral. Table IV-1 provides a few key clinical features to indicate a possible cause that should be included in the differential diagnosis.

TABLE IV–1: SIGNS AND SYMPTOMS	
Signs and Symptoms	*Possible Diagnosis (Specialist)*
Pain at the angle of the mandible brought on by exertion and relieved by rest	Cardiac ischemia owing to coronary artery disease (Internal Medicine/Cardiology/ Oral Medicine)
Severe unilateral pain in the maxilla and orbit associated with autonomic signs; tearing and redness of the eye, runny nose, drooping of the upper eyelid	Cluster headache (Neurology/Oral Medicine)
Headache and facial pain preceded by sensory, motor, or visual phenomena	Vascular/transitional headache (Neurology/Oral Medicine)
Unilateral, brief, sharp, lancinating, severe pain associated with stimulation of specific trigger zones	Trigeminal neuralgia (Neurology, Oral Medicine)
Signs and symptoms of trigeminal neuralgia in a young person (less than 40 yr of age)	Multiple sclerosis (Neurology, Internal Medicine)
Maxillary or midline lower frontal pain with evidence of infection coinciding with the headache; pain may change when the position of the head is changed	Sinusitis (Otolaryngology)

TABLE IV–1: SIGNS AND SYMPTOMS (CONTINUED)	
Signs and Symptoms	*Possible Diagnosis (Specialist)*
Pain from the maxillary first molar and/or second bicuspid when these teeth test vital, are positive to percussion, and demonstrate no rationale for pulpal disease	Sinusitis (Otolaryngology)
Severe, throbbing, temporal pain associated with chewing	Temporal arteritis, vascular pain (Ophthalmology, Rheumatology/Internal Medicine / Oral Medicine)
Pain behavior that is exaggerated or inconsistent with dental periodontal pain; indications of depression, personality disorder, and suicidal thoughts	Psychological disorders (Psychiatry, or Psychology)
Orofacial pain and pain in other body locations of undetermined cause and not responsive to treatment	Chronic pain syndrome (Oral Medicine / Internal Medicine, Rheumatology, Chronic Pain Clinic)
Masticatory muscle pain and dysfunction associated with generalized pain and a nonrestorative sleep pattern	Fibromyalgia (Internal Medicine, Rheumatology/ Oral Medicine, Physical Medicine)
Increasing severe headache associated with nausea, vomiting, and other neurologic symptoms	Intracranial tumor or blood vessel malformation (Neurology, Internal Medicine, Oral Medicine)
Orofacial pain and hearing loss	Acoustic neuroma (Otolaryngology, Neurology)
Pain associated with altered sensation confirmed by objective examination	Trauma or tumor invasion of nerves (Internal Medicine, Otolaryngology, Neurology, Oncology)
Earache, trismus, altered sensation in the distribution of the mandibular nerve	Carcinoma of the infratemporal fossa (Otolaryngology, Oncology)
Episodic pain with discrete swelling occurring just before and during meals	Obstructive sialoadenitis (Otolaryngology, Oral and Maxillofacial Surgery, Oral Medicine)
Localized toothache, no radiographic signs of pulpal pathology, questionable diagnostic test data, and pain not relieved by local anesthesia	Atypical facial pain (Oral Medicine, Endodontics)
Diffuse chronic orofacial pain not confined to neuroanatomic boundaries, unremitting without variation, and no physical findings to identify cause	Atypical facial pain/complex regional pain syndrome (reflex sympathetic dystrophy) (Oral Medicine, Endodontics, Anesthesiology, Chronic Pain Clinic)
Diffuse protracted burning pain not confined to neuroanatomic boundaries and no physical findings	Complex regional pain syndrome (reflex sympathetic dystrophy) (Oral Medicine, Anesthesiology, Chronic Pain Clinic)

PATIENT MANAGEMENT

For the practitioner, referral is usually looked on as a logical step toward a solution. For the patient, the suggestion may be greeted with ambivalence and anxiety. The underlying communication that should guide the discussion is the practitioner's belief that consultation is in the patient's best interest. Patients experiencing pain and suffering urgently request relief. This creates a pressure to try to do everything possible as soon as possible to alleviate pain. It is important to explain that the reason for not immediately starting treatment is the lack of a definite diagnosis and the possibility that inappropriate treatment may cause more problems. In a circumstance in which an odontogenic or periodontal diagnosis cannot be established, the most valuable contribution the dentist can make is to recommend against treatment until a diagnosis is established.

PATIENT RECORDS AND INFORMATION

The patient should be advised that all relevant information pertaining to the problem will be forwarded to the specialist in advance of the appointment. Record the date of the appointment in the patient's chart. This will ensure that all records, including radiographs, laboratory tests, and correspondence, will be forwarded and received prior to the visit. Patients are often anxious about whether previous records have reached the consultant and may make a point of asking if records have been received. Noting the appointment date also facilitates a timely follow-up telephone call. To facilitate the referral, a release may be provided for the patient's signature, and this signed release may be forwarded to the consultant.

It may be helpful to provide a preprinted patient-doctor agreement concerning the sharing of information with other health professionals. Different jurisdictions may have different regulations concerning confidentiality and should be consulted to ensure compliance. This can be presented and discussed prior to the consultation visit or when discussion of the patient's case with other health care professionals may be necessary.

INFORMATION ABOUT THE SPECIALIST
Arranging the Appointment
Making the appointment before the patient leaves the office is likely to increase patient attendance for the consultation appointment.

Correspondence
A formal request for the consultation should be made. This should be in written form, identifying the patient, the reason for the referral, the history of present illness and medical history, previous treatment, and any other relevant information.

Patient Contact after the Consultation
If possible, the patient should be called after the consultation visit. This will give the patient the opportunity to discuss any concerns about the consultation and will provide the practitioner with feedback.

The patient should be advised that the practitioner will continue to provide any dental treatment that is necessary.

Patients are most likely to have a long-term relationship with the GP, and they will appreciate the GP's continued involvement. It is also reassuring to the patient to know that the GP is available to discuss any concerns or issues that arise during the diagnostic process or treatment.

INFORMATION HELPFUL FOR THE CONSULTANT
- Relevant information about the referring clinician: name, address, e-mail address, facsimile and telephone numbers
- Relevant descriptive information about the patient: name, age, address, telephone number, cultural background, and gender
- Statement of the condition for which the patient is being referred, tentative diagnoses or concerns
- Relevant information regarding the problem, including a history of the present illness, medical history, previous test results, and diagnostic imaging examinations
- Specific requests that might include particular blood studies, diagnostic tests, or therapeutic trials

CONCLUSION
Successful referral occurs when the patient understands that the recommendation is in his or her best interest. The consultant's assessment may well prove negative, but ruling out certain disorders is often necessary as part of the diagnostic process. An important part of any practice is the network of individuals with other skills who can be relied on to help solve difficult diagnostic and treatment problems. Following patients' experiences, reviewing reports and discussing cases with specialists provides the basis for evaluating the care provided and is also educational. This ongoing communication contributes to better patient care. Patients acknowledge and trust the practitioner who is able to evaluate a problem and identify another health professional who might best manage the problem. In this context, the referral builds trust and strengthens the dentist's relationship with the patient.

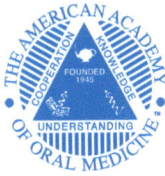

References

- Alexander WN. 1991. *Practical oral medicine and clinical laboratory diagnosis for the general dentist.* Minneapolis (MN): Burgess/Alpha Editions.

- American Academy of Craniomandibular Disorders, McNeill C, editor. 1993. *Temporomandibular disorders: guidelines for evaluation, diagnosis, and management.* 2nd ed. Chicago: Quintessence.

- American Academy of Orofacial Pain. De Leeuw R, Klasser GD, editors. 2013. *Orofacial Pain Guidelines For Assessment, Diagnosis, And Management.* Fifth Edition: Chicago; Quintessence.

- American Dental Association Council on Scientific Affairs. 2006. "The use of dental radiographs. Update and recommendations." *J Am Dent Assoc* 137: 1304–12.

- Austin BD, Shupe SM. 1993. "The role of physical therapy in recovery after temporomandibular joint surgery." *J Oral Maxillofac Surg* 51: 495–8.

- Balciunas BA, Siegel MA, Grace EG. 1992. "A clinical approach to the diagnosis of facial pain." *Dent Clin North Am* 36: 987–1000.

- Banford A, Remick RA, Blasberg B. 1986. "Tardive dyskinesia: an unrecognized cause of oral facial pain." *Oral Surg Oral Med Oral Pathol* 61: 570–2.

- Barasch A, Elad S, Altman A, et al. 2006. "Antimicrobials, mucosal coating agents, anesthetics, analgesics, and nutritional supplements for alimentary tract mucositis." *Support Care Cancer* 14: 528–32.

- Barker F, Jannetta P, Bissonette D, et al. 1996. "The long term outcome of microvascular decompression for trigeminal neuralgia." *N Engl J Med* 334: 1077–83.

- Barker GJ, Epstein JB, Williams KB, et al. 2005. "Current practice and knowledge of oral care for cancer patients: a survey of supportive health care providers." *Support Care Cancer* 13: 32–41.

- Benoleil R, Epstein J, Eliav E, et al. 2007. "Orofacial pain in cancer: part I — mechanisms." *J Dent Res* 86 (Jun): 491–505.

- Blasberg B, Chalmers A. 1989. "Temporomandibular pain and dysfunction and generalized musculoskeletal disorders." *J. Rheumatol* 15: 87–90.

- Blasberg B, Remick RA, Miles JE. 1983. "The psychiatric referral in dentistry: indications and mechanics." *Oral Surg Oral Med Oral Pathol* 56: 368–71.

- Borowski B, Benhamou E, Pico JL, et al. 1994. "Prevention of oral mucositis in patients treated with high-dose chemotherapy and bone marrow transplantation: a randomized controlled trial comparing two protocols of dental care." *Eur J Cancer B Oral Oncol* 30: 93–7.

- Bouquot JE, Roberg AM, Person P, Christian J. 1992. "Neuralgia-inducing cavitational osteonecrosis (NICO)." *Oral Surg Oral Med Oral Pathol* 73: 307–20.

- Brooks SL, Brand JW, Gibbs SJ, et al. 1997. "Imaging of the temporomandibular joint. A position paper of the American Academy of Oral and Maxillofacial Radiology." *Oral Surg Oral Med Oral Pathol Oral Radiol Endod* 83: 609–18.

- Brown CR, Funt L, Chase P, et al. 1995. "Position paper: the dentist's role as a pain specialist in the diagnosis and treatment of head, face, and neck pain." *Am J Pain Manag* 5: 79.

- Brown RS, Bottomley WK. 1990. "On the utilization and mechanism of tricyclic antidepressants in the treatment of chronic facial pain." *Anesth Prog* 37: 223–9.

- Brown RS, Bottomley WK. 1990. "On the utilization and mechanism of tricyclic antidepressants in the treatment of chronic facial pain." *Anes Prog* 37: 223–9.

- Brown RS, Farquharson AA, Sam FE, Reid E. 2006. "A retrospective evaluation of 56 patients with oral burning and limited clinical findings." *Gen Dent* 54: 267–71.

- Burchiel KJ, Johans TJ, Ochoa J. 1993. "The surgical treatment of painful traumatic neuromas." *J Neurosurg* 78: 714–9.

- Callender KI, Brooks SL. 1996. "The usefulness of tomography in the evaluation of patients with temporomandibular disorders: a retrospective clinical study." *Oral Surg Oral Med Oral Pathol Oral Radiol Endod* 81: 710–9.

- Canavan D, Graff-Radford SB, Gratt BM. 1994. "Traumatic dysesthesia of the trigeminal nerve." *J Orofac Pain* 8: 391–5.

- Carlson CR, Miller CS, Reid KL. 2000. "Psychosocial profiles of patients with burning mouth syndrome." *J Orofac Pain* 14: 59–64.

- Carroll LJ, Ferrari R, Cassidy JD. "Reduced or painful jaw movement after collision-related injuries; a populatin-based study." 2007. *JADA* 138: 86–93.

- Clark GT, Minakuchi H. 2006. "Oral appliances." In *Temporomandibular disorders*, edited by Laskin DM, Green CS, Hylander WL, 377–90. Chicago: Quintessence.

- Clark GT, Ram S. 2007. "Four oral motor disorders: bruxism, dystonia, dyskinesia and druginduced dystonic extrapyramidal reactions." *Dent Clin North Am* 51: 225–43.

- Clark GT. 2006. "Persistent orodental pain, atypical odontalgia, and phantom tooth pain: when are they neuropathic disorders?" *J Calif Dent Assoc* 34: 599–609.

- Cohen SG, Quinn PD. 1988. "Facial trismus and myofascial pain associated with infections and malignant disease: report of five cases." *Oral Surg Oral Med Oral Pathol* 65: 538–44.

- Cooper BC, Cooper DL. 1991. "Multidisciplinary approach to the differential diagnosis of facial head and neck pain." *J Prosthet Dent* 66: 72–8.

- Currey TA, Dalsania J. 1991. "Treatment for herpes zoster opthalmicus: stellate ganglion block as a treatment for acute pain and prevention of post-herpetic neuralgia." *Ann Ophthalmol* 23:188–9.

- Danhauer SC, Miller CS, Rhodus NL, Carlson CR. 2002. "Impact of criteria-based diagnosis of burning mouth syndrome on treatment outcome." *J Orofac Pain* 16: 305–11.

- Dao TT, Lavigne GJ, Charbonneau A, et al. 1994. "The efficacy of oral splints in the treatment of myofascial pain of the jaw muscles: a controlled clinical trial." *Pain* 56: 85–94.

- Dolwick MF. 1997. "The role of temporomandibular joint surgery in the treatment of patients with internal derangement." *Oral Surg Oral Med Oral Pathol Oral Radiol Endod* 83: 150–5.

- Dube C, Rompre PH, Manzini C, et al. 2004. "Quantitative polygraphic controlled study on efficacy and safety of oral splint devices in tooth-grinding subjects." *J Dent Res* 83: 398–403.

- Dworkin SF, Burgess JA. 1987. "Orofacial pain of psychogenic origin: current concepts and classification." *J Am Dent Assoc* 115: 565–71.

- Dworkin SF, Sherman J, Mancl L, et al. 2002. "Reliability, validity, and clinical utility of the research diagnostic criteria for Temporomandibular Disorders Axis II Scales: depression, nonspecific physical symptoms, and graded chronic pain." *J Orofac Pain* 16: 207–20.

- Dworkin SF. 1995. "Behavioral characteristics of chronic temporomandibular disorders: diagnosis and assessment." In: *Temporomandibular disorders and related pain conditions*, edited by Sessle BJ, Bryant PS, Dionne RA, 175–92. Seattle, WA: IASP Press.

- Eli I, Kleinhauz M, Baht R, Littner M. 1994. "Antecedents of burning mouth syndrome (glossodynia) — recent life events." *J Dent Res* 73: 567–72.

- Eliasson S, Isacsson G. 1992. "Radiographic signs of temporomandibular disorders to predict outcome of treatment." *J Craniomandib Disord Facial Oral Pain* 6: 281–7.

- Epstein JB, Elad S, Eliav E, Jurevic R, Benoliel R. 2007. "Orofacial pain in cancer: part II—clinical perspectives and management." *J Dent Res* 86 (Jun): 506–18.

- Epstein JB, Epstein JD, Epstein MS, et al. 2006. "Oral doxepin rinse: the analgesic effect and duration of pain reduction in patients with oral mucositis due to cancer therapy." *Anesth Analg* 103: 465–70.

- Epstein JB, Klasser GD. 2006 "Emerging approaches for prophylaxis and management of oropharyngeal mucositis in cancer therapy." *Expert Opin Emerg Drugs* 11: 353–73.

- Epstein JB, Marcoe JH. 1994. "Topical application of capsaicin for treatment of oral neuropathic pain and trigeminal neuralgia." *Oral Surg Oral Med Oral Pathol* 77: 135–40.

- Epstein JB, Schubert MM. 2004. "Managing pain in mucositis." *Semin Oncol Nurs* 20: 30–7.

- Epstein JB, Stewart KH. 1993. "Radiation therapy and pain in patients with head and neck cancer." *Eur J Cancer B Oral Oncol* 29: 191–9.

- Epstein JB. 1990. "Neurologic diseases: dental correlations." In: *Internal medicine for dentistry*, edited by Rose L and Kaye D, 755–70. St. Louis: CV Mosby.

- Feinmann C, Newton-John T. 2004 "Psychiatric and psychological management considerations associated with nerve damage and neuropathic trigerminal pain." *J Orofac Pain* 18: 360–4.

- Frazier CH, Russell EC. Neuralgia of the face. 1924. "An analysis of 754 cases with relation to pain and other sensory phenomenon before and after operation." *Arch Neurol Psychiatry* 11: 557–63.

- Frediani F. 2005. "Pharmacological therapy of atypical facial pain: actuality and perspective." *Neurol Sci* 26 Suppl 2: 92– 4.

- Fricton JR, Dubner R, editors. 1994. *Orofacial pain and temporomandibular disorders*. Philadelphia: Lippincott, Williams & Wilkins.

- Friedlander AH, Runyon C. 1990. "Temporal arteritis." *Oral Surg Oral Med Oral Pathol* 69: 317–21.

- Gangarosa LP, Mahan PE, Ciarlone AE. 1991. "Pharmacologic management of temporomandibular joint disorders and chronic head and neck pain." *J Craniomandib Pract* 9: 328–38.

- Gatchel RJ, Garofalo JP, Ellis E, Holt C. 1996. "Major psychological disorders in acute and chronic TMD." *J Am Dent Assoc* 127: 1365–74.

- Glass EG, McGlynn FD, Glaros AG. 1991. "A survey of treatments for myofascial pain dysfunction." *Cranio* 9: 165–8.

- Gorsky M, Silverman S, Chinn H. 1991. "Clinical characteristics and management outcome in burning mouth syndrome: an open study of 130 patients." *Oral Surg Oral Med Oral Pathol* 72: 192–5.

- Goulet JP, Lund JP, Montplaisir JY, Lavigne GJ. 1993. "Daily clenching, nocturnal bruxism, and stress and their association with TMD symptoms." *J Orofac Pain* 7: 120.

- Graff-Radford SB, Goldberg WK. 1986. "Atypical odontalgia." *Calif Dent Assoc J* 14: 27–32.

- Greenberg MS, Cohen SG, McKittrick JC, Cassileth PA. 1982. "The oral flora as a source of septicemia in patients with acute leukemia." *Oral Surg Oral Med Oral Pathol* 53: 32–6.

- Greene CS, Obrez A. 2015. "Treating temporomandibular disorders with permanent mandibular repositioning: is it medically necessary?" *Oral Surg Oral Med Oral Pathol Oral Radiol* 119: 489-98.

- Gregg JM. 1990. "Studies of traumatic neuralgias in the maxillofacial region: surgical pathology and neural mechanisms." *J Oral Maxillofac Surg* 48: 228–37.

- Gremeau-Richard C, Woda A, Navez ML, et al. 2004. "Topical clonazepam in stomatodynia: a randomized – placebo – controlled study." *Pain* 108: 51–7.

- Gremillion HA, Waxenberg LB, Myers CD, Benson MB. 2003. "Psychological considerations in the diagnosis and management of temporomandibular disorders and orofacial pain." *Gen Dent* 51: 168–72.

- Grushka M, Epstein JB, Gorsky M. 2003. "Burning mouth syndrome and other oral sensory disorders: a unifying hypothesis." *Pain Res Manag* 8: 133–5.

- Grushka M. 1987. "Clinical features of burning mouth syndrome." *Oral Surg Oral Med Oral Pathol* 63: 30–6.

- Gruska M, Epstein J, Mott A. 1998. "An open-label, dose escalation pilot study of the effect of clonazepam in burning mouth syndrome." *Oral Surg Oral Med Oral Pathol Oral Radiol Endod* 86: 557–61.

- Hansson LG, Hansson T, Petersson A. 1983. "A comparison between clinical and radiologic findings in 259 temporomandibular joint patients." *J Prosthet Dent* 50: 89–94.

- Hargitai IA. 2004. "Comorbid findings in an orofacial pain population." *Oral Surg Oral Med Oral Pathol Oral Radiol Endod* 97: 450

- Hickey AJ, Toth BB, Lindquist SB. 1982. "Effect of intravenous hyperalimentation and oral care on the development of oral stomatitis during cancer chemotherapy." *J Prosthet Dent* 47: 188–93.

- Hinderstein B, Baughman D, Lewis V. 1997. "Efficacy of splint therapy in a private dental practice." *Oral Surg Oral Med Oral Pathol Oral Radiol Endod* 84: 163.

- Huynh N, Lavigne GJ, Lanfranchi PA, et al. 2006. "The effect of 2 sympatholytic medications – propranolol and clonidine – on sleep bruxism: experimental randomized controlled studies." *Sleep* 29: 307–16.

- Ikeda T, Nishigawa K, Konda K, et al. 1996. "Criteria for the detection of sleep-associated bruxism in humans." *J Orofac Pain* 10: 270–82.

- International Association for the Study of Pain. 1995. *Classification of chronic pain: descriptions of chronic pain syndromes and definitions of pain terms.* 2nd ed. Seattle, WA: IASP Press.

- Inturrisis CE. 1989. "Management of cancer pain: pharmacology and principles of management." *Cancer* 63: 2308–20.

- Jacobson AL, Donlon WC, editors. 1990. *Headache and facial pain.* New York: Raven Press.

- Kandel EJ, Schwartz JH, Jessell TM, editors. 2000. *Principles of neural science.* 4th ed. New York: Elsevier.

- Keith DA, Glyman ML. 1991. "Infratemporal space pathosis mimicking TMJ disorders." *J Am Dent Assoc* 122: 59–60.

- Khan OA. 1998. "Gabapentin relieves trigeminal neuralgia in multiple sclerosis patients." *Neurology* 51: 611–4.

- Klasser GD, Balasurbramariam R, Epstein J. 2007. "Topical review-connective tissue diseases: orofacial manifestations including pain." *J Orofac Pain* 21: 171–84.

- Konzelman JL, Herman WW. 1996. "Chronic orofacial sensory disorders." In: *Clark's clinical dentistry.* Vol. 1. edited by Hardin JF, 1–6. St. Louis: Mosby-Yearbook.

- Korszun A, Hinderstein B, Wong M. 1996. "Comorbidity of depression with chronic facial pain and temporomandibular disorders." *Oral Surg Oral Med Oral Pathol Oral Radiol Endod* 82: 496–500.

- Kreiner M, Betancor E, Clark GT. 2001 "Occlusal stabilization appliance. Evidence of their efficacy." *J Am Dent Assoc* 132: 770–7.

- Lamey PJ, Lamb AB. 1988. "Prospective study of aetiological factors in burning mouth syndrome." *BMJ* 296: 1234–6.

- Laskin DM, Green CS, Hylander WL, editors. 2006. *Temporomandibular disorders.* Chicago: Quintessence.

- Lavigne GJ, Lobbezoo F, Montplaisir JY. 1995. "The genesis of rhythmic masticatory muscle activity and bruxism during sleep." In: *Brain and oral functions,* edited by Morimoto T, Matsuya T, Takada K, 249–55. Amsterdam: Elsevier.

- Lavigne GJ, Montplaisir JY. 1995. "Bruxism: epidemiology, diagnosis, pathophysiology and pharmacology." In: *Orofacial and temporomandibular disorders,* edited by Fricton JR, Dubner R, 387–404. New York: Raven Press.

- Lavigne GJ, Rompré PH, Montplaisir JY, Lobbezoo F. 1997. "Motor activity in sleep bruxism with concomitant jaw muscle pain: a retrospective pilot study." *Eur J Oral Sci* 105: 92–5.

- Lavigne GJ, Rompré PH, Montplaisir JY. 1996. "Sleep bruxism: validity of diagnostic criteria and motor variables in a controlled polysomnographic study." *J Dent Res* 75: 546–52.

- Lavigne GJ. Kato T, Kolta A, Sessle BJ. 2003. "Neurobiological mechanisms involved in sleep bruxism." *Crit Rev Oral Biol Med* 14: 30–46.

- Levitt SR, McKinney MW, Lundeen TF. 1988. "The TMJ Scale: cross validation and reliability studies." *Cranio* 6: 17–25.

- Levy RA, Smith DL. 1989. "Clinical differences among nonsteroidal antiinflammatory drugs: implications for therapeutic substitution in ambulatory patients." *DICP* 23: 76–85.

- Lewit K. 1981. "Muskelfaxilitations und Inhibitions — Techhniken in der Manuellen Medizin. Teil II. Postisometrische Muskelrelaxation." *Man Med* 19: 12–22.

- Lindquist SF, Hickey AJ, Drane JB. 1979. "Effect of oral hygiene on stomatitis in patients receiving cancer chemotherapy." *J Prosthet Dent* 40: 312–4.

- Lobbezoo F, Thu Thon M, Rémillard G, et al. 1996. "Relationship between sleep, neck muscle activity, and pain in cervical dystonia." *Can J Neurol Sci* 23: 285–90.

- Lotaif AC, Mitrirattanakul S, Clark GT. 2006. "Orofacial muscle pain: new advances in concept and therapy." *J Calif Dent Assoc* 34:625–30.

- Lund JP, Lavigne GJ, Dubner R, Sessle BJ, editors. 2001. *Orofacial pain. From basic science to clinical management. The transfer of knowledge in pain research to education.* Chicago: Quintessence Publishing Co, Inc.

- Mahan PE, Alling CC III. 1991. *Facial pain.* 3rd ed. Philadelphia: Lea & Febiger.

- Marbach JJ, Lennon MC, Dohrenwend BP. 1988. "Candidate risk factors for temporomandibular pain and dysfunction syndrome:psychosocial, health behavior, physical illness and injury." *Pain* 34: 139–51.

- McNeill C. 1992. *Current controversies in temporomandibular disorders.* Carol Stream (IL): Quintessence.

- McQuay H, Carrol D, Jadad A, et al. 1995. "Anticonvulsant drugs for management of pain: a systematic review." *BMJ* 311: 1047–52.

- McQuay H, Tramer M, Nye B, et al. A systematic review of antidepressants in neuropathic pain. Pain 1996;68:217– 27.

- Mejersjö C, Hollender L. 1984. "Radiography of the temporomandibular joint in female patients with TMJ pain or dysfunction. A seven year follow-up." *Acta Radiol Diagn (Stockh)* 25: 169–76.

- Melzack R, Wall PD. 1965. "Pain mechanisms: a new theory." *Science* 150: 971–9.

- Merskey H, Bogduk N, editors. 1994. *Classification of chronic pain: descriptions of chronic pain syndromes and definitions of pain terms.* 2nd ed. Seattle, WA: International Association for the Study of Pain Press.

- Modi BJ, Knab B, Feldman LE, et al. 2005. "Review of current treatment practices for carcinoma of the head and neck." *Expert Opin Pharmacother* 6: 1143–55.

- Mohammed SE, Christensen LV, Penchas J. 1997. "A randomized double-blind clinical trial of the effect of amitriptyline on nocturnal masseteric motor activity (sleep bruxism)." *J Craniomandib Pract* 15: 326–32.

- Moldofsky H. 1989. "Sleep and fibrositis syndrome." *Rheum Dis Clin North Am* 15: 91–103.

- Mongini F, Rota E, Deregibus A, et al. 2005. "A comparitive analysis of personality profile and muscle tenderness between chronic migraine and chronic tension-type headache." *Neurol Sci* 26: 203–7.

- Mongini F. 1999. *Headache and facial pain.* Stuttgart: Thieme.

- Monks R. 1994. "Psychotropic drugs." In: *Textbook of pain,* edited by Wall PD and Melzack R, 963–89. Edinburgh: Churchill Livingstone.

- Mott AE, Grushka M, Sessle BJ. 1993. "Diagnosis and management of taste disorders and burning mouth syndrome." *Dent Clin North Am* 37: 33–71.

- Nilner M, Petersson A. 1995. "Clinical and radiological findings related to treatment outcome in patients with temporomandibular disorders." *Dentomaxillofac Radiol* 24: 128–31.

- Okeson JP, editor. 1996. *Orofacial pain: guidelines for assessment diagnosis, and management.* Chicago: Quintessence.

- Okeson JP. 2005. *Bell's orofacial pains.* 6th ed. Chicago: Quintessence.

- Okeson JP. 1993. *Management of temporomandibular disorder and occlusion.* 3rd ed. St. Louis: Mosby-Year Book.

- Ohrbach R, Gonzalez Y, List T, Michelotti A, Schiffman E. 2013. "Diagnostic Criteria for Temporomandibular Disorders (DC/TMD)" *Clinical Examination Protocol: version 02* June. http://www.rdc-tmdinternational.org.

- Oturai A, Jensen K, Eriksen J, Madsen F. 1996. "Neurosurgery for trigeminal neuralgia: comparison of alcohol block, neurectomy, and radiofrequency coagulation." *Clin J Pain* 12: 311–5.

- Peterson DE. 1990. "Pretreatment strategies for infection; prevention in chemotherapy patients." *NCI Monogr* 9: 61–71.

- Pullinger AG, White SC. 1995. "Efficacy of TMJ radiographs in terms of expected versus actual findings." *Oral Surg Oral Med Oral Pathol Oral Radiol Endod* 79: 367–74.

- Raja SN, Treede RD, Davis KD, Campbell JN. 1991. "Systemic alpha-adrenergic blockade with phentolamine: a diagnostic test for sympathetically maintained pain." *Anesthesiology* 74: 691–8.

- Ram S, Kumar SK, Clark GT. 2006. "Using oral medications, infusions and injections for differential diagnosis of orofacial pain." *J Calif Dent Assoc* 34: 645–54.

- Reid KI and Greene CS. 2013. Review article – "Diagnosis and treatment of temporomandibular disorders: an ethical analysis of current practices." *Journal of Oral Rehabilitation* 40: 546-561.

- Remick RA, Blasberg B, Barton JS, et al. 1983. "Ineffective dental and surgical treatment associated with atypical facial pain." *Oral Surg Oral Med Oral Pathol* 55: 355–8.

- Remick RA, Blasberg B, Campos PE,Miles JE. 1983. "Psychiatric disorders associated with atypical facial pain." *Can J Psychiatry* 28: 178–81.

- Richlin DM. 1991. "Nonnarcotic analgesics and tricyclic antidepressants for the treatment of chronic nonmalignant pain." *Mt Sinai J Med* 58: 221–8.

- Rubenstein EB, Peterson DE, Schubert M, et al. 2004. "Mucositis Study Section of the Multinational Assocation for Supportive Care in Cancer. International Society for Oral Oncology. Clinical practice guidelines for the prevention and treatment of cancer therapy-induced oral and gastrointestinal mucositis." *Cancer* 100 Suppl 1: 2026–46.

- Sale H, Isberg A. 2007. "Delayed temporomandibular joint pain and dysfunction induced by whiplash trauma." *JADA* 138 (8): 1084–91.

- Sarnat BG, Laskin DM, editors. 1992. *The temporomandibular joint: a biological basis for clinical practice.* 4th ed. Philadelphia: WB Saunders.

- Shintaku W, Encico R, Broussard J, Clark GT. 2006. "Diagnostic imaging for chronic orofacial pain, maxillofacial osseous and soft tissue pathology and temporomandibular disorders." *J Calif Dent Assoc* 34: 633–44.

- Scrivani SJ, Matthews ES, Maciewicz RJ. 2005. "Trigeminal neuralgia." *Oral Surg Oral Med Oral Pathol Oral Radiol Endod* 100: 527-38

- Schiffman et al. 2014. "Diagnostic Criteria for Temporomandibular Disorders (DC/TMD) for Clinical and Research Applications: Recommendations of the International RDC/TMD Consortium Network and Orofacial Pain Special Interest Group." *Journal of Oral & Facial Pain and Headache* 28: 1:6-27.

- Ship JA, Grushka M, Lipton JA, et al. 1995. "Burning mouth syndrome: an update." *J Am Dent Assoc* 126: 842–53.

- Silverman S Jr, Eversole LR, Truelove EL, editors. 2002. *Essentials of oral medicine.* Hamilton (ON): BC Decker Inc.

- Simons DG, Travell JG. 1999. *Simons and Travell's myofascial pain and dysfunction: the trigger point manual.* Volume 1. Baltimore: Williams & Wilkins.

- Singer E, Dionne R. 1997. "A controlled evaluation of ibuprofen and diazepam for chronic orofacial muscle pain." *J Orofac Pain* 11: 139–46.

- Sonis S, Kunz A. 1988. "Impact of improved dental services on the frequency of oral complications of cancer therapy for patients with non-head-and-neck malignancies." *Oral Surg Oral Med Oral Pathol* 65: 19–23.

- Stanton-Hicks M, Janig W, Hassenbusch S, et al. 1995. "Reflex sympathetic dystrophy: changing concepts and taxonomy." *Pain* 63: 127–33.

- Travell JG, Simons DG. 1983. *Myofascial pain: a trigger point manual.* Baltimore: Williams & Wilkins.

- Truelove E, Huggins KH, Mancl L, Dworkin SF. 2006. "The efficacy of traditional, low-cost and nonsplint therapies for temporomandibular disorder: a randomized controlled trial." *J Am Dent Assoc* 137: 1099–107.

- Truelove E. 2004. "Management issues of neuropathic trigeminal pain from a dental perspective." *J Orofac Pain* 18: 374–80.

- Turner JA, Dworkin SF. 2004. "Screening for psychosocial risk factors in patients with chronic orofacial pain: recent advances." *J Am Dent Assoc* 135: 1119–25.

- Von Korff M, Ormel J, Keefe FJ, Dworkin SF. 1992. "Grading the severity of chronic pain." *Pain* 50: 133–49.

- Wassell RW, Adams N, Kelly PJ. 2006 "The treatment of temporomandibular disorders with stabilizing splints in general practice: one-year follow-up." *J Am Dent Assoc* 137: 1089–98.

- Weissmann G. 1987. "Pathogenesis of inflammation. Effects of the pharmacological manipulation of arachidonic acid metabolism on the cytological response to inflammatory stimuli." *Drugs* 33: 28–37.

- White SC, Pullinger AG. 1995. "Impact of TMJ radiographs on clinician decision making." *Oral Surg Oral Med Oral Pathol Oral Radiol Endod* 79: 375–81.

- Woda A, Navez ML, Picard P, et al. 1998. "A possible therapeutuic solution for stomatodynia (burning mouth syndrome)." *J Orofac Pain* 12: 272–8.

- Woda A, Tubert-Jeannin S, Bouhassira D, et al. 2005. "Towards a new taxonomy of idiopathic orofacial pain." *Pain* 116: 396–406.

- Zakrzewska JM, Chaundry Z, Nurimikko T, et al. 1997. "Lamotrigine in refractory trigeminal neuralgia: results from a double-blind placebo controlled crossover trial." *Pain* 73: 223–30.

- Zakrzewska JM, Harrison SD, editors. 2002. *Assessment and management of orofacial pain.* London: Elsevier.

- Zarcone VP. Sleep hygiene. 1994. In: *Principles and practice of sleep medicine*, edited by Kryger MH, Roth T, and Demet WC, 542–6. Philadelphia: WB Saunders.

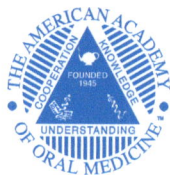

The American Academy of Oral Medicine
2150 N. 107th St., Suite 205
Seattle, Washington 98133
PHONE: (206) 209-5279 · EMAIL: info@aaom.com

Application for AAOM Membership

ELIGIBILITY FOR MEMBERSHIP

1. Nominee for **Regular Membership** shall be a graduate of an accredited Dental School or Medicine School and shall be a member of his/her representative National Society and shall pursue special interest or accomplishment in the field of Oral Medicine.

2. Nominee for **Affiliate Membership** (student) shall be a graduate of an accredited Dental or Medical School and shall be a member of his/her representative National Society and currently in training in a Postdoctoral program.

3. Nominee for **Student Membership** shall be a student currently enrolled in a pre-doctoral program in an accredited dental or medical school. Students are those seeking a DDS, DMD or MD degree.

4. The fiscal year for dues starts January 1.

5. After acceptance into the Academy, Active Membership dues are paid annually and include a subscription to ORAL SURGERY, ORAL MEDICINE, ORAL PATHOLOGY, ORAL RADIOLOGY, and ENDODONTOLOGY.

6. Please see the AAOM website for more membership information and how to apply: www.aaom.com.

www.ingramcontent.com/pod-product-compliance
Lightning Source LLC
Chambersburg PA
CBHW041451210326
41599CB00004B/216